TONI
MY STORY

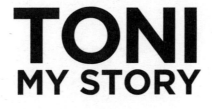

TONI
MY STORY

THE RAGS-TO-RICHES STORY OF TONI&GUY, 'HAIRDRESSER TO THE WORLD'

TONI MASCOLO
WITH STAFFORD HILDRED

JOHN BLAKE

Published by
John Blake Publishing Limited
3 Bramber Court, 2 Bramber Road
London W14 9PB

www.johnblakepublishing.co.uk

www.facebook.com/johnblakebooks ◼
twitter.com/jblakebooks ◼

First published in hardback in 2015

ISBN: 978-1-78418-116-1

British Library Cataloguing-in-Publication Data:

A catalogue record for this book is available from the British Library.

Design by www.envydesign.co.uk

Printed in Great Britain by CPI Group (UK) Ltd

1 3 5 7 9 10 8 6 4 2

Papers used by John Blake Publishing are natural, recyclable products
made from wood grown in sustainable forests. The manufacturing processes
conform to the environmental regulations of the country of origin.

Every attempt has been made to contact the relevant copyright-holders,
but some were unobtainable. We would be grateful if the appropriate
people could contact us.

CONTENTS

CHAPTER ONE

SCAFATI:
EARLY DAYS

Of all the countless times and places there are to be born, somehow I managed to arrive right in the middle of the greatest conflict our planet has ever seen. World War Two was raging savagely in many regions across the globe when I arrived on 6 May 1942 and the place of my birth, the sleepy little town of Scafati, near Pompeii in southern Italy, was soon to find itself right on the frontline.

Happily, I was not remotely aware of any of the military action and horrendous loss of life. I was a much-loved year-old toddler taking his first unsteady steps when the war came right through Scafati. The first major Allied assault on the mainland of Europe began with the landings at nearby Salerno in September 1943. British troops fought very bravely and the Germans were forced to retreat. The bridge over the River Sarno in Scafati became an important early objective and, with the help of courageous local partisans, the British captured the bridge just before the Germans were able to blow it up and so prevented the likely devastation of my hometown.

Today a plaque in Scafati commemorates the action and there is a real warmth of feeling for the British people, which I have many, many different reasons of my own for sharing. But as a young child growing up in a loving family, I was barely aware of the horrors of war. My father, Franco, was the local barber, a position of some importance in our close-knit society. My mother, Maria, was caring and kind and beautiful. As a little boy I was firmly convinced she was the most wonderful woman in the world, and as I grew up this was not an opinion that ever changed.

My mother was a member of the wealthy Gallo family, who were merchants who sold wine, tomatoes and all sorts of other produce. They had their own flour-mill and lived in Messigno, a village just outside Pompeii. The family included mathematicians and other distinguished professionals and belonged to an elite branch of society. If you had a flour-mill in Italy, you had power. Clearly, they were people of substance.

My father's family, on the other hand, comprised mere hair-dressers and entertainers. My grandfather had owned a barber's shop in Torre Annunziata, a town west of Pompeii, but he died very young. On the day of his funeral thieves raided the shop and stole everything, even the mirrors. My father had a very difficult upbringing and never had much of an education. He was just nine years old when he lost his father; he and his siblings were adopted by an aunt who was married to another barber. The fate of my grandmother is to this day unknown to me. I later learned that the family more or less disowned her after she refused to have anything to do with her own children after her husband's death. My father never ever spoke about his mother to me. As I was growing up I knew my great-aunt and great-uncle as my grandparents. They were very sweet and I loved them dearly.

Back in those days a barber's shop in Italy was not just somewhere people went to have their hair cut. It was also the place where medical emergencies were handled; it was almost like a hospital. The barber's wife was commonly a midwife who could help to deliver babies, while the barber himself was often called upon to stitch wounds, pull out rotten teeth and, in extreme cases, even to perform amputations. It was because they had sharp razors and they knew how to use them. The barber was the only man with the tools – very sharp, fine blades – to perform such jobs, and the expertise in using those tools. As time went on, the doctors and the hospitals took over these tasks and then the life of the barber changed. He became more of a comic and an entertainer as well as a hairdresser. But the barber's shop remained a very important place at the heart of the community.

Still devastated by the early death of his father, the nine-year-old Franco was soon hard at work shaving customers and helping out in his uncle's barber's shop. He had a desperately difficult time as a boy but the move to his aunt's did have its own happy outcome. His new home was near to where my mother lived, which led to the first meeting. They quickly became friends and in due course fell in love. My mother's family certainly did not welcome the idea of a match between the barber's offspring and their beautiful young daughter Maria, the youngest of their eight children. The Gallo family believed she could do much better than the boy from the barber's shop. My father was a great romantic and he used to serenade her as the relationship developed. After it became clear that there was a strong attraction between young Maria and Franco, her brothers took direct action to derail the relationship –

and put bars across the windows of her bedroom so that my father could not get in!

But other considerations became more important as war engulfed Europe. The old order changed for good, and love proved stronger than social distinctions. My future parents were eventually able to overcome all opposition and after a carefully chaperoned courtship they were married. Life together was happy but never easy. Franco and Maria worked hard to make a success of his new hairdressing salon in Scafati. Times were often tough, especially when my mother's first baby, a little girl, was stillborn. For a young couple keen to start a family this was heartbreaking, especially since my mother had really wanted a daughter. Later, my father was conscripted into the Italian Army and my mother had to strive hard to keep the salon running while he was away. My arrival must have further increased her workload, but my earliest recollections are of a sublimely happy couple and a household full of life and laughter.

Our home was a flat by the side of the river, not far from the salon. Scafati has some 50,000 occupants today but the population was much smaller when I was growing up there. The town was nevertheless busy and full of small businesses trying to make a living. There was a town hall, a splendid church, a primary school, a secondary school and two cinemas. Scafati even had two railway stations: the state railway station, with trains running to Rome and Milan, and the local station, where trains ran around Mount Vesuvius. Scafati is only about two kilometres from Pompeii and you could travel there by tram. When I was a boy Pompeii and Scafati were separated by glorious open countryside, which has long since been built on and covered with roads, houses, shops and factories. Vesuvius was not such a popular tourist attraction then as it is today. In fact it is hard to believe that when I was young there were so few foreigners that, once, when a black man visited, people were paying money just to look at him! No one had ever seen a coloured person in the flesh so he became a little sideshow at the ruins. There were few visitors and Scafati was the sort of community where all the people knew each other. Everyone lived in flats and there always seemed to be lots of family and friends around.

Although it was very busy and our home was small I did manage to find a private place where I could keep my most precious things safe. There used to be a big wardrobe across a corner window and I was small enough to creep underneath and the little space behind was my secret hideaway. Underneath the wardrobe there was a ledge and my treasures were hidden there. I used to keep all my coins and football pictures safe there. From a young age I was keen on conserving things. I always liked to save things and hated to waste anything, and that has never changed.

My earliest recollections are mainly warm and joyful though I remember at night being frightened of the darkness outside the big door to our apartment. There were no lights in the passage so I used to run very fast, scared that ghosts were lurking in the blackness.

The flats seemed enormous to me as a boy, and all sorts of people were our neighbours. You could have the plumber living next to the hairdresser and the lawyer or the doctor nearby. The main road from Germany that goes all the way down to Sicily came right through the town so it was always busy and full of life. I remember when I was very small there were people on horses and donkeys pulling carts, but soon cars and lorries took over the road. The policemen and the guards from the town hall used to shout at everybody and it was bustling but very friendly. I had lots of friends and relations and from a young age we children used to roam freely round the town.

My real first name is Giuseppe – the name Toni did not come into my life until much later. About eighteen months after I was born my brother Gaetano arrived. He was to become known as Guy, but again, not until many years later. When we were small there was enough of an age gap to make quite a difference. My brother was much more like my father than I was. Gaetano was quite flashy even as a young boy. He was always wanting this and wanting that, always demanding toys. Whenever we went out he was forever demanding something, while I would always be more careful about asking for money. I used to think anxiously to myself: *Maybe they can't afford it*. Even as a young child I was very cautious: I did not want to put any pressure on my mum and dad. I didn't want to put pressure on anybody, but particularly not my parents.

Gaetano was very attractive, even as a young boy. He had long hair, which was styled in waves and ringlets, and he often looked like a little girl (I think this was partly because my mother really yearned for a daughter). We were close as young brothers but we were very different. There is an old photograph of me aged six sitting on a step and looking very angry. My parents had gone with the two of us boys to a professional photographer and I felt it was not fair that Gaetano was getting all the attention and seemed to be the subject of all of the photographs. The younger one is always the favourite and Gaetano was always very spoilt. Being a Taurus, I absorb a lot of things and then I snap and lose my temper. That time I became really angry because I felt I was being ignored, so my parents got the photographer to take a picture of me. You can see how upset I was!

My father went away to Naples to learn how to do perms and soon he was in great demand. He was busy at the salon but also at weekends when there were weddings to prepare for. In those days the bride would want a perm, as would many of the guests. When I was a little boy, I recall, people used to knock on the door as early as five o'clock in the morning so he could do their hair. He was a very clever, artistic man.

Long before I knew where England was I used to hear my father speaking highly of that country. From his experiences in the war he used to say that when the English bombed a bridge they would do so by dropping one bomb on the bridge and causing no other destruction, so it was not just Scafati they had saved. But, my father said, when the Americans came they would bomb the bridge and everything 300 yards on either side, causing widespread damage.

My mother was so kind and caring; she always watched out for us but I could be wilful and difficult at times and I remember I learned my lesson the hard way. I think I was about four years old and my mother was washing me in a part of the kitchen we used for washing ourselves. She placed me on a chair and told me not to move as it was not very stable. I was messing about and she again warned: 'Sit still and don't move from that chair or you will hit your head.' What did I do? Of course I moved and cracked my head open! I still have the mark today. I had to be taken down to the chemist's and have stitches put in.

Our neighbours were our friends and as a child I was often running in and out of other people's flats. The family next door were called Pastore and the father was the stationmaster of the town's state-run railway. It was quite a big powerful job and they had a bigger place than us. They had six or seven rooms while we had only two. The father would always come home to eat his meal and then he would have his apple. He made quite a performance of peeling it slowly and carefully, almost like clockwork. They had three daughters and the second one got married to a captain in the army. It was a fantastic wedding that created lots of excitement in the family and soon afterwards she was expecting a baby and again there was so much joy and happiness. Sadly, she died giving birth. Everyone was desperately upset. Tragic events like that stay in your mind forever.

The Pastore family came from Naples and were middle class. The head of the family was bald and had a little tummy; he was a bit too friendly towards my mother. She was always pushing him away, saying: 'Go away and leave me alone! Don't touch me.' I don't think anything serious happened – he just thought he could take advantage of a young married woman when her husband was not around. Even at a very young age I was very aware of what was going on around me; maybe sometimes I took too much notice. Sometimes perhaps a clear memory is not such a good thing. I can remember every bloody little thing!

Lots of friends and relations lived around us so it was a wonderful community to grow up in. Most people did not have a great deal of money and some were very poor but everyone had plenty of food. Even the poorest people had food in their cellar. They might be short of cash but they always had tomatoes, artichokes, potatoes, prosciutto, salami and other delicious things to eat. I remember going to my aunt's in the country and marvelling at all the different types of food. There were no fridges in those days but there was a well near my aunt's house to keep the food cool, including fresh melon and all sorts of fruit, as well as wine. Every Sunday lunch was a precious time spent together as a family, and to enjoy cold wine and fruit on a hot Sunday afternoon was most refreshing. There was not a great deal of meat but they used a lot of vegetables: pasta with beans, broccoli and cauliflower. In those days nothing was ever wasted. If there was any spaghetti left over they would fry it with a couple of eggs and make a kind of pizza. After my uncle came home from work I would go to the field with him; he used a spring to irrigate his field and the water tasted so fresh and beautiful. My brothers and I used to help pick fruit and tomatoes and we just loved being outside in the sunshine.

It was a very healthy way of life – I can't remember ever feeling ill. We had such a nutritious diet and we spent so much time outside building up our immune systems, unlike the children of today who seem to be indoors all of the time. Nowadays I think that is one of our big problems: everything is protected by disinfectant so our immune systems are not naturally built up as well as in years ago.

From the age of six I attended school. My mother took me on the first day but after that I went every day by myself. It was only a few hundred yards over the bridge from our flat. At school you had to pass every exam before you could go up to the next year. In Italy, the rule was that it was no good going up to the next stage if you did not know all the basics – you had to know the two and three times tables before you went on to anything more difficult. They brought in outside teachers to test the pupils because the school believed that it had to be a proper test (they did not want any teachers' favourites being waved through). You had to be good at everything – it was no good doing well in history and geography if you were hopeless at maths. I enjoyed lessons and found I was a quick learner and so I did very well. I had help from the age of four at pre-school so I skipped the first year in primary school and then at six I joined the second year, therefore I was able to enter the local secondary school a bit earlier.

Mind you, I was much better at maths than I was at some of the more creative subjects. I remember being completely stumped when we were asked to come up with an essay about trees. 'Well, there is a beautiful tree with a trunk and leaves and branches,' I wrote. Then I pretty well ran out of anything to say. My teacher was horrified and she said: 'What are you doing? Haven't you got any imagination? All you seem to like is numbers!' She was dead right there.

As young boys we used to swim in the River Sarno, near where it goes into the sea. We had some fantastic days playing there. There was a real innocence about growing up in Scafati in those days. As a child you could walk anywhere without fear of being molested. It always felt safe and I think it *was* safe. There were no problems, apart from sometimes when you went to the cinema. Some of the guys there would try and touch your leg if you weren't careful. My mother always warned me to be very careful where I sat.

I did as I was told and I always liked going to the cinema, but I enjoyed being outdoors even more. We used to go often to Messigno, where my Aunty Rosa lived, which meant a magnificent walk through the countryside alongside the River Sarno that took roughly about an hour. I had an older cousin, Franchino, who lived there and he was very good at woodwork. He kindly made us a little cart and fixed it so the goat could pull us along in it, like a miniature horse and carriage. We would sit there laughing as the goat did all the work; as young kids we thought it was hilarious. I spent a lot of time with my cousin. He was lots and lots of fun and we had some great times together. Often we would go for a swim in the crystal-clear waters of the River Sarno. You could even see little fish swimming around; it was so clean and beautiful. It is quite unbelievable today, with all of the tomato factories – it's a complete mess, unrecognisable from the good old days.

There was always plenty of good food to eat in the countryside – I loved it! Now and then they would kill a pig, which made for a great feast. Once the knife got stuck in the creature's throat when they were killing it and it ran off with the knife sticking out. It was incredible. Eventually they got hold of him and it was a wonderful party. They used to fry all the blood with lots and lots of onions. We had pork chops on the barbecue and it was great fun.

I also used to spend a lot of time with my Zia (Aunt) Elvira and Zio (Uncle) Placido, who lived in the countryside just outside Scafati. Often I spent time with my older cousin, Alfonso. He was passionate about game shooting and I remember sometimes staying until the small hours helping him to refill cartridges and put everything in the proper place. I felt extremely useful and was pleased to be able to help him. Early in the morning I used to accompany him through the countryside where he was doing his shooting. For me it was an amazing magical time and I enjoyed the lovely walks and nice fresh fruit that you could pick; I always looked forward to that. And I remember coming home totally satisfied with my achievement.

However, I could be quite naughty as well. There were lots of fiestas in the countryside and once when I was with my cousin Franchino there was a kind of fair with stalls. There were some horses tied to the sweets stall and I started messing around, causing them to bolt and the stall was pulled over. There were sweets everywhere and everything went flying. I didn't do it on purpose but I knew I might be in trouble. When people began to ask what had happened I pointed to this rather slow-looking local boy with thick glasses and said: 'It was him.' So he was in trouble and not me. Later, I felt guilty and wished I hadn't done it.

But in general I was not naughty – I left that to others. The one time when I was the one who got into trouble was when I was about eleven and desperately wanted to go and watch a film in a new style called Cinemascope. It was being screened about fifteen kilometres away and I told my mother I was going to go with some friends to see it. It meant coming back home quite late and she said firmly: 'You are not going *anywhere*.' She emphasised the last word so I knew she meant business as she very rarely spoke sharply to me. I pleaded that I would be back home by 10.30 but she said, 'No,' and I knew she meant it.

However, I was now determined so I decided to go anyway. I cannot recall much about the film but I can remember in detail what happened when I returned. When I got home I sneaked into the flat as quietly as I could. My bed was close to the entrance so I slid in as softly as possible. Just as I was starting to relax and beginning to think I had got away with it my mother burst in, extremely angry and very upset with me. She told me how wrong I had been to go out without permission and she hit me with a slipper, even though I could see she did not really want to hurt me. My mother would never hurt a fly, let alone her own son, and they were very gentle smacks.

I realised then that she must have been desperately worried and I felt very guilty. She must have been terrified that something awful would happen to me and she just wanted to get all that out of her system. Looking back afterwards I thought what a dreadful boy I had been and I did feel very ashamed. I adored my mother and I never wanted to hurt her.

I don't believe I was ever that badly behaved but if ever there was a time I could have gone slightly off the rails it was when I was eleven or twelve years old. That was when my snooker playing and gambling were in danger of getting a little out of control. I used to go out and gamble and play all sorts of games for money; I would have bets with other kids and even go into bars and play snooker for money with bigger boys. You had to put some money down and stand up for yourself but I was never afraid of that.

I don't remember experiencing any fear apart from the time when my cousin Vito, who was eleven years older than me, unexpectedly visited the bar. I had a lot of respect for him and he was teaching me after school. Of course I was embarrassed and humiliated in his presence – even though he didn't say a word, just gave me a deep look.

I never risked a lot of money at my gambling but I was good at table football and I think perhaps I was on the verge of getting involved with the wrong sort of people. But Vito saw the danger and he quickly fished me out. He said I was mixing with bad people, who were a bad influence and I listened to him. When you are a kid you need some guidance and Vito was very wise and he steered me back on to the right track. Always a great inspiration to me, he went on to become a professor of mathematics. He was my mentor and even today, all these years later, we are still very close.

One terrifying experience was when another older cousin, Alfonso, took me for a tour in a car to see the beautiful resorts of Positano and Amalfi. They were stunning but most of the time I was too frightened to look as there were then no barriers in place along the coast road and some of the sheer drops were absolutely terrifying. We sped along in one of the first Fiat automobiles at 100 kilometres an hour. It was my own fault – I wanted to try everything.

My father was a remarkable man. He was gifted and charming and devoted to my mother but in spite of all his talents he was much too relaxed and easy-going to be a very successful businessman. Early on he made a small fortune as a hairdresser and at one point he had enough money to buy several properties and he could have made himself very secure. Instead of being prudent and doing that he kept the cash – following the war the money was devalued and became worthless. It was a shattering experience, but my father was not an educated man. He didn't know how to invest in something safe and sensible; he had the money and he was very generous to lots of people while he had it.

After it was gone he just shrugged and went back to work in the salon. Because of his undoubted talents he was in great demand as a hairdresser and he made a lot of money again; he had a trade and a talent that lots of people wanted. He was an eternal optimist and with all the women of the town competing for his services he was like a star. Franco the hairdresser! Everybody knew him, not only in Scafati but also in Pompeii and all the other towns around. He was very good, very experienced, because he was the first one to put personality into hairdressing in that way. And he made another fortune. But he was always very generous and as soon as he had money he spent it. He would take all of his staff to one of the top restaurants and paid for all the pizza, beer and wine they could consume.

My father always believed in living life to the full. A larger-than-life character, he was quite irrepressible when things were going well. Sometimes if he was busy he would work until he dropped, but once he had made enough money he liked to stop work and do something else for a while. Even as a young boy I was a worrier and most of all I worried about my mother. She was so gentle and innocent that sometimes her feelings were lost in my father's enthusiasms. Father was also a bit of a gambler – he loved to play cards with his friends at the men's clubs while my mother was left at home. She would never enter one of those places, so when I was about eight or nine when the time got to about 10 o'clock at night I would be sent to bring him home. I would go in and the place would be full of smoke and laughter. There might be twenty tables of men sitting round, playing poker. I used to stand behind my father and say that he had to come home. Usually he would laugh and say: 'One more game.' Always it was more than just the one more game and eventually I would almost have to pull him out. But my father would just laugh – he was a make-money, spend-money kind of guy.

His fame grew even more in 1953 when he entered the Italian hairdressing championship in Naples. And he took me with him to the finals. He was always very confident that his famous 'artichoke' style – with hair wound round like the vegetable – would impress the judges and he was right. He won the coveted title of Best in Italy and became an overnight hero in the hairdressing world. At the finals he told me to go and introduce myself to the President. At the time I was very shy and I thought to myself that I really didn't need to be pushed towards the limelight. I was only eleven years old, a very serious, studious boy. So I went and shook hands but I was very embarrassed. I wasn't really interested in hairdressing; I just used to help my father winding perms and shampoos at busy times, like Christmas. I had no thought then that I would ever work properly as a hairdresser – I just enjoyed helping out in the salon for a little bit of cash.

At school I was always the youngest in the class because I was one year in front. I loved much of the schoolwork, especially maths, but it was the writings of the great Roman leader Julius Caesar that particularly fascinated me. I was able to read about 80 per cent of them in the original Latin after studying it for almost four years and I became tremendously impressed by Caesar's own accounts, particularly of his time invading Great Britain. For me the details of the battles and how he devised his strategies were quite compelling. The way Caesar took advantage of the landscape, and always tried to attack from higher ground, was brilliant. I was enthralled by his descriptions of the foot-soldiers of the Roman Army in their impeccable uniforms, marching with a very strong beat, creating a powerful sound that could destroy bridges and tree-houses, inspiring fear in the enemy. His use of different tactics was amazing, though I never came close to imagining what a help everything I learned from Caesar would be to me in later life. I was very excited by him and obviously extremely proud of the Roman Empire; it gave me some feeling of confidence and understanding of power. I just couldn't put the books down and I never forgot them.

My world was very stable and happy and I was beginning to think that my progress at school might mean I could go to university and perhaps become a lawyer or an accountant. But that was before my impulsive father revealed to the family that 'Best in Italy' was no longer enough for him; he intended to strike out for the big-time.

We were heading for London.

CHAPTER TWO

THE CAPITAL
OF THE WORLD

The sudden news that the whole family was to move to London was unbelievably exciting to an impressionable fourteen-year-old. To me it meant that we were all going to live in the most glamorous of cities: London, surely was the capital of the world? Practical problems like young children switching countries as well as schools, sorting out the hairdressing business in Scafati and the awkward fact that none of the Mascolos could speak any English somehow seemed sublimely unimportant as my father enthusiastically spelt out his plans for the future.

The idea for our sudden migration across Europe came from an Italian hairdresser called Biagio, who had established himself in London. Back on a visit to his home country, he sparked my father's interest in a move to England when he asked him provocatively what he was doing, as a winner of the Best in Italy award, working 'in this little village' of Scafati. Biagio boasted that he had an exclusive salon in London's stylish Knightsbridge district where his client list included all the leading high-society ladies, from queens and duchesses to film stars such as Gina Lollobrigida and Sophia Loren. He added that he had his own coffee bar and even enthused that he flew to work in his own helicopter, which he loved to land in the conveniently placed Hyde Park.

My father was hooked. Always a great optimist, he had complete confidence in his skills as a hairdresser. I remember him saying: 'It is better to live one day as a lion than one hundred years as a sheep!' He agreed to go to London to check out this captivating new opportunity. On arrival he soon discovered that, while the helicopter existed only in Biagio's imagination, the salon was real enough and so too were the possibilities for the future. He enjoyed working in Biagio's salon and even though he spoke no English he found no problem in communication as the clients soon warmed to his easy charm. His next task was to convince my mother of the wisdom of the move.

My father brought her over and they stayed in stylish Kensington for a couple of months. He showed her the sights and took her to Harrods, where she sampled 'sandwiches' for the first time. My mother loved London and quickly agreed to the move – in any case her family had already advised her that under no circumstances should she let my father go on his own. Although a happily married man, he always had an eye for the ladies. My mother was not well-educated but she was a brilliant home-maker, who was trained to do sewing and cooking to a very high standard. She knew perfectly well that if my father came to England, she and the family would join him there. There were lots of English girls around and she knew her husband. He had a reputation for being very self-confident and flashy, being one of the first men in Scafati to wear a white suit and to ride the latest Italian motorbike made by Ducati. But it was love that motivated my mother: she would have gone after my father wherever he went. If he had said he was going to the moon, she would have happily followed him.

The decision was quickly made and the whole family – that is, my father and mother, myself, my brothers Guy, who was twelve, Bruno, who was eight, and three-year-old Andrea – set off on the uncomfortable three-day train journey to England. In the days before budget airlines it was the only way we could afford to travel, but it was still a thrill. We broke the journey in Milan, where we stayed with one of my dad's former hairdressers. Even that was a big event for me – I had never experienced central heating before.

Eventually we arrived in England and when we got off the Channel ferry at Dover we saw all these neat little houses and everything seemed quite magical. I was used to everyone living in flats and these pretty homes looked amazing. It was just like Disneyland, which had opened in America the previous year. *When we get to London it's going to be amazing. I'll find money on the streets*, I thought. But it wasn't quite like that and I came quickly back down to earth when we arrived in our new home.

My father had clearly pulled out all the stops to show my mother the best possible side of London on her visit but he could not afford to keep up those high standards. That became very clear to us as we explored our new accommodation at Number 12, Gerrard Road, Islington. The house was owned by an Italian couple, who were living in Bedford; the wife was a nurse. They wanted to make some money by renting out rooms. There were five floors, which were all let out to Italians from different parts of northern Italy as well as from Naples, Sicily and Calabria. Every weekend the occupants used to play cards, get into heavy discussions, which soon turned into heated debates, and with all of the different dialects it sometimes sounded utterly chaotic! For a fourteen-year-old it was a very exciting experience.

It was the best part of London for us in one way because it was near the Italian church, where a lot of our country folk used to go. Unfortunately it was a damp basement flat with only a small coal fire to heat it. There was little in the way of modern facilities and no washing machine. My mother had my father and the four of us to take care of, and my youngest brother Anthony was soon on the way. The Islington of the 1950s was a world away from the gentrified area of today. Back then it was down-at-heel, bomb-damaged and downright depressing. I can't imagine what my mother must have felt as the grim reality of Gerrard Road sank in, yet I always remember her with a smile on her face – my father's famous charm must have been working overtime.

Although I knew my mother's heart must have really sunk, I was overjoyed to be in London. I hardly gave a thought to the dingy flat because I was so excited to be in this thrilling city. Everything was so new I felt I had really arrived in the world. I remember just marvelling at simple things like the big red buses criss-crossing the city; I used to watch the huge queues near our home in Islington and marvel at the masses of people getting on board for their journey to the West End. The signs on the bus for famous destinations like Leicester Square and Piccadilly were somehow exhilarating in themselves. After a lifetime in a peaceful backwater I felt as if I had come to the hub of everything; I couldn't have been happier, especially when travelling on the Tube. I used to write letters back to Italy explaining with great enthusiasm that you could go down under the ground in one place and then come up anywhere you wanted! I had never seen anything like it before. Our local station was Angel and you could go down underground and end your journey miles away, wherever you wanted to be. To me it was just fabulous. London seemed to be a place that had everything. I loved exploring the city.

The people seemed polite and friendly. Everything was very ordered and disciplined. I felt at home very soon in London. In those days if you got off a bus before you had had the chance to pay for your ticket, you would leave the money on the seat for the conductor. It was unbelievable to me; in Italy that would have been inconceivable (we would always try to dodge the conductor on the tram). In London bread and milk were delivered and left untouched outside people's houses. I even saw a big box of money that had been left by the newspaperman unguarded outside a pub in central London while he was inside having a drink, and no one would touch it. Back home that would have been unthinkable. The English policemen too were completely different from their Italian counterparts. In London police officers were polite and very helpful if you asked them directions, while back in Scafati they would have boxed your ears if you had bothered them with your silly questions.

I felt stimulated and alive, and from the first moment I loved London. But of course not everything about my new life was easy. I soon found that going to school was anything but the happy experience it had been in Italy. The leaving age was fifteen so I still had to attend. Because at first I didn't speak a word of English I had to attend the Italian School that was under the church in nearby Clerkenwell Road. It was totally different from going to school in Italy. I was shocked to find that instead of the order and discipline I had been accustomed to in Scafati there was a lot of noise and wild behaviour. One male teacher took the roll-call every morning, which was a new experience to me, and took quite a long time. Then the next minute, after everyone had said they were present, he was selling chocolate and drinks! Everyone seemed to have half a pint of milk and biscuits. Then there would be reading for perhaps ten or fifteen minutes before it was time for football and other games.

Many of the lessons were not very academic. We did a bit of woodwork, which was interesting, and quite a lot of sport, which hardly featured at school in Italy.

Some of the children were well-behaved and studied hard but others could not even read or write and were a little wild. The English boy who sat next to me could not even write his own name. He scrawled like I had done years before as a little boy of four with the nuns. There was a lot of bad behaviour too. There was no teacher with anything like the iron control of the elderly lady who had ruled the classroom so firmly in Italy. One day some of the kids ambushed a teacher and completely stripped him of all his clothes, down to his pants. He was a guy in his forties and it was eight or nine fourteen- or fifteen-year-olds who set on him – I think they thought he had picked on one or two of them. I had never seen anything like it in Italy and I was totally shocked by this outrageous attack and kept out of it. Back home the standards of respect and behaviour were much higher. And in Italy there was a great deterrent that if you were badly behaved then you might be kept down a class and not be able to leave school. In the Italian School in England there was no deterrent, really. It was very casual and relaxed, very take-it-or-leave-it.

One of the ringleaders was a little boy with a big knife and he once waved it threateningly in front of me and said: 'I'm in charge. I'm the boss.' If he was trying to frighten me, it didn't work. I didn't argue but I was not scared and showed it and so they didn't pick on me at all because I was very definite and didn't get involved. Most of the time I was very happy. It was a great, great time of my life – I loved England and the English people from the day I arrived. Perhaps the only thing I disliked was the school dinners. In Italy we didn't have school dinners because we went home and did our homework in the afternoon. To be honest, I was a bit disillusioned by the school. I thought, *If this is the capital of the world, surely the education should be better?* Of course in those days I had no knowledge of places like Oxford or Cambridge, or of the country's top public schools. I was very puzzled as I thought English schools would be even better run than those in my home country. But this was inner London, with children of a wide range of abilities who came from many different parts of the world, and later I realised that in the majority of other English schools such behaviour would not have been tolerated.

Coming to London gave me a feeling of reality that I loved. I knew it was a great city and pretty soon I didn't want to live anywhere else. But there were new dangers to be faced. Life was very different from what I was used to, back in Italy. The streets of Scafati had always seemed totally safe to me but the streets of London were a different matter. The late 1950s saw the rise of the gangs of teddy boys who were often at the centre of trouble. Screenings of the 1956 film *Rock Around the Clock* featuring Bill Haley and the Comets sparked teddy-boy riots in cinemas all over the country in the year of our arrival. Although I tried hard not to show any fear, I was concerned by the gangs, and was very wary. I was always extremely nervous in the early days of living in Gerrard Road that there would be a gang of teddy boys behind me when I was going to catch the bus. They could be violent and dangerous and there were several alarming skirmishes in a little square near the high street in Islington.

It was hard for all the family to come to terms with our new life. My father worked long hours with Biagio and after he had left the salon he often worked in the evenings as well, tending to the hair of some of the numerous young Italian nurses who had come over to work in the big London hospitals. My mother was always very busy, dealing with a new home in a new country and my younger brothers were adapting to their new schools and making friends. While we were managing to cope one way or another, it was clear that one of our biggest problems was that none of us could speak more than a few words of English.

Frustrated that I could not communicate properly, I decided to learn the language properly. So I found myself a teacher, a young man in Battersea. He had an office job and was not really a teacher but gave lessons in his spare time. I used to travel on the 137 bus to his little basement flat, where he had to put coins in the meter to keep warm, in those days quite a commonplace practice in the UK. I'd go on my own for a couple of hours in the evenings and I soon picked up the basics. He was a really nice man and he taught me a lot. I looked forward to my visits because I was learning so much and he was a congenial person. His upper-class accent seemed to give him a lot of confidence and I thought that I would love to be like him. My accent was pretty awful but at least I could understand and speak English. Naturally, I then became the translator for the whole family.

That was a real help because while my father could handle his job in the salon well enough, my mother found shopping for food very difficult. English people seemed to prepare meals in completely different ways to the methods she was used to in Italy.

I remember how shocked I was the first time someone said to me: 'I'm going to have my tea.' I said: 'Why? Are you sick?'

And when I discovered that he was going to eat mashed potato and sausages I was even more surprised. The food sounded very strange, but tea? 'Surely you're going to have a glass of wine with it?' I asked, but for most English people at that time, wine did not seem to exist. I slowly realised that the vast majority of the population was working class and it was only the small minority of upper-class people who drank château-produced wine and knew about brandy, whisky and all the upmarket drinks. In Italy even though we didn't have any money we still ate and drank very well, with our pizza and pasta and good wine and Peroni beer. If you had gone into the cellars of poor people in Italy in the 1950s you would always have found prosciutto, salami, tomatoes, artichokes, aubergines and good potatoes. Although they did not have a lot of money, they had supplies of good food. In England I soon discovered this was not the case; often the cupboard really was bare.

The class system puzzled me too. In Italy there seemed to be warmth and respect between all kinds of people. The local plumber would be friendly with the town's leading lawyer and often they would visit the same restaurant or the same church. In England life seemed more divided by income and background, yet there was straightforwardness about many aspects of life that I preferred. The business of acquiring a new flat in Italy might involve both private recommendations and hefty backhanders, while buying a new home seemed so much simpler in England – as long as you had the money.

Although times were hard we were a happy family and we began to enjoy living in London more and more. I believe the Italians have always had a deep affection for the British, though they tend to think of them as simply English. When I was growing up in Italy there was always a tremendous respect for the people of Britain. My family and friends regarded the British as a people who were very fair, very honest and very sporting. They never really liked the French or the Germans; they always felt the British and the Italians were very similar in many ways.

When I came to London I was impressed by the history of a nation that once had a huge empire covering a large part of the world. Italy was then a comparatively recently unified country but I saw parallels between the Roman Empire and the British Empire. I thought back to Julius Caesar's accounts of his campaigns – which, as I mentioned earlier, I so much enjoyed reading. In my mind I would picture every battle, admiring the way Caesar prepared them right down to the last detail, how, in the end, even if his armies were outnumbered he always emerged triumphant. These were images that never left me and much later they became the base and foundation of my drive to establish and build up my company, Toni & Guy.

My father's shortcomings with the English language did not impede his work greatly. Always smartly dressed and usually with a fresh carnation in his buttonhole and a smile on his face, he was an instant success with Biagio's clients. But he was less than impressed with Biagio himself. It was not just the absence of the promised helicopter, but the fact that the salon owner took time off from work to paint his home. That really confused my dad. As he said: 'Biagio is a bit of an imposter. He's got all this money and then he paints his own house!'

Of course, if my father had not uprooted the family I believe I would probably have continued with my studies, gone to university and then chosen a safe and well-paid career in Scafati as an accountant or a lawyer and my life would have been very different. Before I had settled down I would have loved to have travelled and lived and worked in France and then moved on perhaps to Spain. But as my schooldays came to an end I still very much loved being in London. I only attended the Italian School for a few months. When the summer arrived I was fifteen and I could leave school; my education was over and the real world beckoned. It seemed pretty clear to me that in spite of all my previous big ambitions there really was only one choice of career that seemed open to me: hairdressing. Back in Scafati I had often helped in the salon, washing hair, cleaning up or running errands. Despite the complete absence of any relevant training, my father thought it would be no problem at all for me to follow in his line of work full-time.

He had left Biagio's in Knightsbridge by the time I finished school, to work with a barber called Viccari at 23 Cork Street, Mayfair. The kindly Mr Viccari was running a successful shop just cutting men's hair until my father persuaded him to let him rent a small, unused area, already equipped with three cubicles, for ladies. Soon he established a very wide range of regular clients. Some lived in Mayfair while others travelled from outside London. There were landowners' wives, aristocrats, and there were many younger, local ladies, who were very beautiful and elegant. I later learned that quite a number of these 'local ladies' were working as high-class escort girls who entertained wealthy men. For a young boy who had just left school it was an exotic world.

My father gave all the clients these white gowns to wear and they would go behind curtains to change. He would say to me: 'Don't be shy. Go in.' Sometimes the ladies were still half undressed when I entered. At other times they would have their gowns on and while I was shampooing their hair their buttons would somehow become undone. This was all quite a shock for me at the age of fifteen; it was literally an eye-opener. I also remember practising hair on models in the evening. I absolutely loved doing the razor cut similar to the style Gina Lollobrigida sported, very razored and wispy around the face. I really enjoyed that type of hairdressing and I found it extremely satisfying and rewarding. My father was very flamboyant. He would use a cup, not even a bowl, to mix his tints in – always very easy-going, he was happy to break all the rules under the sun. I had never actually cut a client's hair myself but when the moment came, typically my father threw me in at the deep end.

I was very nervous when my father first asked me to do a lady's hair. He saw my hesitation and said: 'Come on, you have been watching me for weeks. How long does it take to learn? A lifetime!' Of course, looking back, it was a wonderful way to gain confidence. Hairdressing very soon became not so much a job for me, but an enjoyable hobby that paid well.

Mayfair in those days was like an elegant village full of charming and interesting people who all seemed to know each other. There were few cars on the roads and you could park anywhere. I grew to like London even more and my conviction that I was now at the centre of the world grew stronger still. Mr Viccari was a rather extravagant personality, like someone from a comical magazine. Sixty-five, he seemed older and was full of character and experience. He was married to a very middle-class English lady and they lived out in Morden. He kept telling me about his two children, one of whom had become a doctor and the other a dentist; he was very proud. He had worked hard and achieved his dreams. Now preparing for retirement, he was anxious to make as much money as he could before he stepped down. He took a real interest in me and said he wanted to guide and help me for the years to come. He explained that he himself had arrived in England at the age of fifteen and that was why he identified with me so strongly – he talked to me a lot.

Mr Viccari had an impressive client list. The actors Alfred Marks, Christopher Lee, the Fairbanks brothers, and the spy-turned-media personality Malcolm Muggeridge were among his regular customers as were at least two kings, several minor royals, fifteen ambassadors – including the Italian Ambassador – and the hotelier Charles Forte.

Mr Viccari was a kind and well-meaning man but I was not at all happy the day he suddenly suggested to me in the salon that I went over to say 'Hello' to the great Mr Forte. I thought, *I'm not a baby,* but I did as I was told and went up and said: '*Buon giorno*, Mr Forte.' He smiled and said that he hoped my new career would go well and gave me a £1 note. This was when my weekly wage was 15 shillings and 11 pence, so I was impressed.

Many years later I met his son, Rocco Forte, who was with the Italian Ambassador, and I told him of his father's kindness. Rocco was polite but not nearly as gracious as his father and swiftly palmed me off as someone who was a bit of a nuisance.

In fact, I learned a great deal from Mr Viccari, particularly when it came to hanging on to money. Although he was the boss he was not exactly generous. I once saw him having coffee in the nearby Burlington Arcade. As I walked in he was very friendly. I said: 'Ah, Mr Viccari, are you going to buy me a coffee?' I certainly thought he would, as he was the boss. But he said: 'Absolutely not.' And then he explained: 'You are fifteen, I am sixty-five. I am going to retire soon. You are much wealthier than me because you have fifty more years of money-making to run. When you get to my age you will be a lot wealthier than I am, so you should buy *me* a coffee.' I wasn't too impressed by his logic so I didn't buy him that coffee!

He was also very clever at drumming up business during quieter times. I remember him more than once telephoning important clients, including the Italian Ambassador, and saying that he had been unable to sleep properly because he was bothered by the knowledge that the client's hair had not been cut for three weeks. The very thought that his client might not looking his best was disturbing the barber's nights! That was his idea of customer service. Viccari used to tell me: 'You've got to teach your clients how to behave.' But he did not always have the last laugh. As Viccari was approaching retirement he came up with the interesting idea that his clients might like to give him goodbye presents. The quick-witted Mr Muggeridge outsmarted Viccari on this occasion quite comprehensively. Muggeridge, later to become editor of *Punch*, produced a joke worthy of the great magazine. He handed over a cheque for £1 million, correctly signed, yet dated to be cashed in the year 2050!

In those days Viccari used to charge 5 shillings for a haircut and 4 shillings and 6 pence for a shampoo. He used to sit on a stool and chat after he had cut a client's hair. He would mutter under his breath 'Five shillings [which was for the haircut], four and six [or the shampoo] and half a crown [as tip]': then, more loudly, he'd say, 'Twelve shillings please, sir.' The client would usually hand over a £1 note and Viccari would clap the side of his pocket, and in spite of the sound of coins rattling, he would say: 'I don't seem to have any change, sir. Lovely day, isn't it?' He would start brushing the back of his client's jacket and usually the client would say: 'Keep the change.'

This used to really anger his assistant Gordon, a very precise and careful man who used to advise clients that a shampoo was a waste of money. This left him charging just the 5 shillings for a haircut. Unlike his boss he couldn't bring himself to add half a crown as tip, so sometimes he only received a shilling, leaving him distraught about being so much less well paid.

I remember that a tailor who had moved from Savile Row opened up for business next door and quickly became Gordon's client. Gordon could not contain himself. The tailor accepted the advice not to have a shampoo, had his hair cut and handed over 5 shillings and a shilling tip. Gordon held his hand out and said: 'I beg your pardon, sir. I have two daughters who are getting ready to be married and with all due respect, you charge £200 for a suit. I am relying on my tips.' Red-faced with embarrassment, the tailor asked: 'What would you like?' Gordon said: 'A least half a crown,' and amazingly the customer handed over a half-crown tip!

I realised even then that working at Viccari's was part of my hairdressing education. There was never a dull moment. Among the many distinguished clients was the London correspondent of the Italian newspaper, *Corriere della Sera*. He had a very full head of extremely strong and spiky hair. He once came in for a haircut and Viccari feigned great surprise, saying: 'Sir, you haven't been in here for a long time. Look at your hair, it's a real mess!' 'Yes, I've been very busy,' said the client. Viccari began cutting the hair. First, he cut one side and said: 'That is one haircut.' Then he cut the other side and said: 'That is another haircut.' Then he cut the front and the back and announced that was two further haircuts. After he had finished Viccari told the journalist that unfortunately because his hair had been left uncut for so long he had had to perform four haircuts, so the price would be four times 5 shillings – £1. The client was a little bit taken aback but he paid. After he had left

Viccari came over to me and said: 'You've got to learn from me. You've got to teach your clients, they've got to come more often. That's the best way to teach them: charge them more money!'

I was fifteen years old and fascinated by this encounter. Somehow Viccari's behaviour did not seem quite right to me. Then about ten days later the correspondent rang to make another appointment. Viccari was very excited that his client was coming back in less than two weeks. 'I told you,' he said to me. 'You have to teach your clients how to behave.' But the correspondent had the last laugh. When he arrived he sat down and waited for the gown to be put on and then said: 'Ah, Viccari, before you start to cut my hair I recall that the last time I hadn't been here for a long time and you charged me for four haircuts. Today, before you start, I have to say that as I was here only ten days ago I would like just half a haircut!' Viccari did not know what to say and then started laughing louder and louder but this client was delighted that he had been able to teach the barber a lesson.

I loved working at Viccari's. Always there was something interesting going on within the elegant surroundings and often it was pure theatre.

However, there were some sides of Viccari I did not admire. The Italian Ambassador was his favourite customer and Viccari would always insist he would remain Italian all his life. He told the Ambassador that he was helping all the other Italians in London – he was desperate to be awarded an Italian knighthood. Eventually he got his wish, although it was the most junior of the three knighthood awards, the Cavaliere del Lavoro, which in those days had a pension attached. What upset me was that while he professed to support his fellow countrymen I had seen him get very angry several times with Italians who had come into the salon. Viccari would yell: 'Go away!'

He was not very helpful to them at all. I was confused; I thought he was dedicated to helping the Italian community.

Viccari was never short of interesting visitors, though. A good-looking young man came in one day and said his name was Vidal Sassoon and that he had a salon round the corner in Bond Street. He was interested in buying Viccari's place. I'm not sure he really had enough money at the time to buy Viccari's but I was still impressed by him. It must have taken a lot of guts just to walk in and ask the owner straight away if he would be prepared to sell. This was the sort of man I might like to try and imitate one day, I thought. I liked his strength and his courage.

★ ★ ★

There was a big improvement on the home front in 1957 when the Mascolo family was able to move out of the cramped flat in Islington and into a big Victorian house in Clapham. We'd only lived for just over a year in Islington before crossing the river to Number 59 Chelsham Road, which was a much better home certainly we needed the space. In April 1957 my youngest brother Anthony was born. There was much celebration but I knew that while my mother was happy that my new brother was healthy and thriving, inside she was desperately disappointed that she still had no daughter. She longed so much for a little girl to complete our family, but she never complained and made sure we got on with making the most of our new surroundings.

What with the move and the new baby, my mother was run off her feet, but then something happened that I would never have imagined in a million years. My Zia Elvira, who at the time was in her late sixties and nearly twenty years older than my mother (who was the youngest of eight children), came to London. Elvira, who had never travelled anywhere for many years, either by train or bus, had finally plucked up the courage to come to London and support her younger sister. This was the same aunty with whom I had spent so many of my early years in Scafati, where she had a small farm and fields with all sorts of animals. Chickens, pigs, cows, donkeys, sheep... you name it, she had it. Her farm was like heaven for a little boy and I enjoyed it immensely. It was something quite magical and to see her again and to witness my mother's beaming smile of delight was wonderful. My mother's happiness was a sight that enriched my heart, a real fairy tale. I was also very excited and happy to explain to my aunt all of the advantages and great things that we could achieve in a much advanced, easy and fair society with a great future for all the family. I was very proud that we had this opportunity in our new country.

We rented half of the house for £5 a week. We had the ground floor, which had a big lounge and another good-sized room at the back, which became my parents' bedroom. My mother was brilliant at making curtains and fitting out the living room; she made everything so beautiful and comfortable. There was another little room, which we rented out to get some extra cash. Downstairs we had a kitchen and a basement with an outside toilet. Then there were another couple of cave-like cellars. We cleaned them up and painted them and made them liveable, though in all honesty I don't think they would qualify as decent accommodation today.

Upstairs lived a chap called David Small and his wife. He worked at Covent Garden market and they soon became good friends of ours. For a time we also put up the Spano family because they had nowhere to live. They were an Italian couple with three children, a son and two daughters, the older of whom, Nella, I became friends with. They stayed for a few months before they were able to move to the house next door. Later, we sublet one room to Enzo and Marion, a young Italian boy and his Scottish girlfriend. She was a bright, lovely girl and he was very handsome and looked a little like Sean Connery. They were friends as well as neighbours so we were all absolutely devastated when Enzo died suddenly from cancer. I'll always remember him.

Just as in Islington, we Italians stuck together a little to try to help each other. The house would always be full of people and at night they would be playing cards and gambling. For a young teenager like me it was very exciting after living in the quiet little town of Scafati. It was like a melting pot of Italians and lots of different accents from our homeland could be heard. At that time all of them seemed to have one thing in mind: to come to England and work for a couple of years and make as much money as they could so as to go back to Italy and buy their home. Pay was much better in England in those days than in Italy.

In fact it was in 1957, the year we moved to Clapham, that the British Prime Minister Sir Harold Macmillan famously said: 'Most of our people have never had it so good!' With more precious living space at last and even a garden to explore, we certainly agreed. But there was more change afoot when my job with Viccari came to an end. He finally sold his salon so both my father and I needed to find somewhere else to earn a living. My father soon found a position with another top Mayfair hairdresser, Renato, in Dover Street. I felt I needed more practical experience and I wanted to get a job where I could rise to the next level without relying on my father. My brother Guy went to work for Renato instead.

I was keen to be independent but it was not so easy. It was 1958 and I was sixteen and for the first time in my young life out of a job. I remember after I had been unemployed for two or three days the feeling of depression it brought was awful. I received no real help or advice; I still couldn't speak English very well. I didn't know what to do so I just decided to go to Stockwell, not far from where we lived, go into the first hairdresser's I saw and ask for a job. It was called Gerrard, and so I walked in and did just that. It was extraordinary. The boss, Braskin, was an outspoken man of Russian-Jewish origin who was a fierce critic of the English for being lazy. He liked the fact I was Italian and thought I would be hard-working. 'Can you cut hair?' he barked at me. I responded yes, I could cut hair, I could perm, I could colour, I could literally do everything and he said: 'OK, you can be the manager.'

I couldn't believe it. One minute I was totally depressed and the next I was absolutely elated. Braskin said he would pay me £2 a week, which was more than double my money from Viccari. And I was in charge of my own salon! It was incredible. Admittedly, it was considerably downmarket from Viccari's elegant establishment as were Braskin's other two shops, in Camberwell and Peckham. But it was a great chance. In spite of the debt I owed him, though, I never really liked him as a person. I particularly disliked his attitude to England and the English people. I loved London from the moment I arrived and when we lived in Islington I started supporting Tottenham Hotspur. Bill Nicholson was then putting together the great team that went on to win the Double and I loved going to White Hart Lane to cheer them on. Today I can still remember the names of every single one of that remarkable team.

But back to the new job, which was a little overwhelming, for while I had watched and learned from my father for a year I was hardly qualified to run a salon. The staff certainly did not think so. The other stylist was a girl called Monica, only a few months younger than myself. She had a big bouffant hairstyle, a tight pencil skirt and a very short temper. When I asked her to do something she replied tartly: 'Do it yourself! Who do you think you are?' From this unpromising beginning we managed to carve out a reasonable working relationship. There was not a large staff, just a promising young chap called Michael Stylianou, who was my apprentice, Monica and a couple of Saturday girls. Between us we would take care of around forty or fifty clients a day. We used to charge 3 shillings and 6 pence for a shampoo and 7 shillings and 6 pence for a permanent wave. Remarkably, the business appeared to be making money.

My new boss had a highly unconventional technique for increasing the income. Every now and again I would arrive for work and find the back door wide open and various things thrown around on the floor, such as tints and shampoo bottles. It looked as if there had been a burglary and my boss would make a rare personal appearance to telephone the police and report a break-in. A kindly local policeman would come and investigate, my boss would offer him a 'nice cup of tea, officer' and then he would tell the policeman about the imaginary robbery. I presume Braskin would then have made an insurance claim, which would provide a useful boost to his income. To me it all seemed very strange and so very funny, like a small drama.

But life always has a way of springing surprises and it was soon after we moved to Chelsham Road and while I was working in Stockwell that I first encountered racial prejudice. I was never a great success with the ladies, though sometimes I would go dancing and find a nice partner. The first girl I hit it off with was from the same street. There were only about three cars in Chelsham Road at that time and her father was one of the car owners. The young girl, whose name I'm afraid I can't recall, and I were nervously kissing each other in the churchyard for a minute or so. Then she pulled away and said: 'Oh! I can't see you any more.' I was very surprised as we seemed to be getting on so well and I couldn't understand why she was dumping me so quickly. She just added: 'I'm not allowed to go with Italians.' I didn't ask why and to be honest it didn't bother me that much – I just thought it was a little ironic for I liked just about everything about England. I knew there were feelings against Italians but I didn't take any notice of them. I used to go to evening classes and some of the other foreign students would criticise England and the English, which made me really angry. 'Why do you come to this country if you don't like England?' I would say to them.

My love life was anything but chequered, but after being rejected on racial grounds I went out with the nice young Italian girl whose family was living with us. Nella was a lovely girl. Everything was quite formal in those days and I went to ask her father if I could ask Nella, who was only fourteen, out. He was very pleased as he could see I was a hard-working young chap. At the back of my mind I thought I should settle down and have a family, even though Nella and I hardly knew each other. As it turned out, her brother, who had been my friend, started being very jealous and obstructive and in the end our relationship just fizzled out.

Meanwhile, my father had taken many of his faithful clients with him when he went to work for the elderly Renato, who was a famous hairdresser with cups and awards to prove it. Renato had once employed a promising young apprentice whose name was Raimondo Pietro Carlo Bessone. Renato told my father the story of the time when Raimondo, a good-looking guy whose skill as a hairdresser was matched by his confidence as a businessman, was eighteen and wanted to open his own salon. Raimondo went to him and suggested they open a new salon together. The idea appealed to Renato, who suggested a 50–50 partnership, but Raimondo insisted he wanted 51 per cent of the business for himself and that upset Renato. Suddenly his young apprentice was telling him he wanted to be boss! Renato told Raimondo to go away and do it his own way. That's exactly what he did and so Raimondo Bessone became 'Teasy-Weasy' Raymond, one of the most successful hairdressers Britain has ever seen, with a string of racehorses to match his collection of salons.

They were exciting times and although I was only young, I soon settled into the responsibility of being the salon manager but at the back of my mind was always my desire to earn extra money so that I could buy a house for my mother. Some nights I would even go into the West End and earn an extra fiver for a few hours washing dishes. Then my father came up with another money-making scheme: he had some contacts who helped him rent another house in Mount Pleasant, at the back of Clerkenwell. He knew if we could get it spruced up then we could sublet it to make a good profit. It was a little house with four floors and I decided to take a week off and do the painting and decorating. By then I had passed my driving test and helped my father to buy our first car, an Austin Cambridge. I will never forget its registration number was 540AXW and I was so proud to be able to drive myself around. It's hard to believe that in those days it was a pleasure to drive around London! I motored over and painted and papered the place from top to bottom. When I had finished I felt a great sense of achievement and my father rented it out. I think he was paying £2 and 10 shillings a week and taking in £10 or £12.

For a young man I suppose I was always very careful with money.

I used to save £1 a week from my wages and tips from Viccari so after two years I had £104 exactly in the post office. I was very consistent and I suppose a little nostalgic for my original home. When I was still seventeen I went on a trip back to Italy. For the first time I had two weeks off, so with my friend Antonio Juliano in his large and lumbering Vauxhall Cresta, I set off to return to Scafati for a holiday. Antonio was from Naples – he was the young man who looked after the salon in Scafati the first time my father came over to London. As we undertook the long drive I was really looking forward to seeing my hometown again. When we arrived I went to see my aunt and said: 'I'm a millionaire,' because I had £104. This was quite a lot of money in Italy and I asked what I could do for her.

I enjoyed seeing my aunt but in other ways it was a very disappointing trip because all of my friends from school seemed to have gone. I was seventeen, almost eighteen, and most of them were a little bit older and they had all left Scafati. Some had joined the army and others had gone to Argentina or to the United States or Canada so there was almost no one I knew there. I felt I had no more friends and no more ties in the town where I was born and brought up. It was very sad, I felt quite awful. *I haven't got any real friends in England either but I have no choice, I have to make a life in England*, I thought to myself. I knew I couldn't go back and carry on with my studies. Yet although I have raised my family and built my business in England, I know that I am truly Italian and that is where I will retire one day.

★   ★   ★

When I came back from Italy I knew I needed to get a better job. My brother Guy had taken over from me at Gerrard. He was the same age as Michael Stylianou, my former apprentice, and he was experiencing the same sort of management problems that I had encountered. Michael found it hard to accept my brother as his new boss. In fact, he responded to one early work instruction to do something with the blunt retort: 'Why don't you do it yourself? Are you paralysed?'

I went into central London for an interview with Robert Fielding, one of the hairdressing chains. I did the hair of two models and they were delighted with my work, but I didn't get the job. I was a bit disappointed and decided they must have wanted someone with better presence or looks. There was, however, a vacancy working for a Mr Lorenzo, who had an upmarket salon in Victoria Street. My father, who was still at Renato's, had noticed the owner was Italian and said he would come with me. I was still a little shy in those days, but even so I really didn't want my father along. At first Lorenzo said to my father: 'He looks too young.' He said to me: 'You should grow a moustache.' I was not very keen on that idea and Lorenzo was clearly not very keen on me. But my father was insistent and told Lorenzo: 'He is brilliant, give him a chance.' My father kept talking and eventually Lorenzo gave me a job. He said my pay would be £8 a week. I thought he was joking – this was four times what I had recently been earning.

Lorenzo also employed a man called Mr Paul and his sister-in-law, Clara. Clara was the receptionist, and used to do everything else, later becoming PA to Mr Lorenzo, whereas Mr Paul had previously worked chopping trees down! Mr Paul had been through the hairdressing training school Morris Master Class and had learned back-combing and other different techniques. Because I was by now quite experienced as a hairdresser I used back-brushing, which was quicker. He thought back-combing was better and advised me to follow his way, which he thought was the quickest technique but I disagreed.

One day I saw Mr Paul sneakily watching me in the mirror so he could learn my back-brushing techniques – I was leaving him behind so he had decided to follow me. He later took a liking to me and was always giving me advice, trying to direct me and prepare me for my future. We had many discussions following on from this that were very beneficial to me.

Lorenzo was an elderly man but he still had plenty of energy and he kept his eye on everything. If he saw a client looking as if she did not quite have the patience to wait her turn he would scream: 'Grab her!' before she had time to head for the door. The first time he did it was quite unnerving. He was equally demanding if you were working alongside him. If he thought you were working too slowly, he would bellow, 'Come on!' to get his message across. Time really was money to Lorenzo, and he never wanted to waste it but he also knew a great deal about making money, as I was about to learn.

After I had been there for two or three weeks and he saw that I was doing quite well, I was earning £8 a week plus 10 per cent commission. Lorenzo then said: 'If you take £35 in a week, you get £1 bonus, £45 one more pound. £55 one more pound, £65 one more pound.' Then he stopped and said: 'Well, I told Paolino and I tell you as well, after £65 we will split it 50–50 on the money you bring in, but no one has ever achieved £65 before.'

I worked hard and started to build up my clients and after three or four weeks I reached £35. So I got £1 bonus. Things went well and soon I was earning around £12.50 a week. That was a good wage. Civil servants were earning around £12 to £20 a week in those days. It was quite a lot of money and for me it was tax-free.

That's what Lorenzo paid me and he put down he paid the tax on some of the money that he paid me, although he just paid out of his pocket in cash.

We started work at eight o'clock in the morning and did a bunch of clients. Then we had a little break, a sandwich or something, and then at 11.30 or 11.45 we started getting busy through lunchtime. We worked hard to do as many clients as we could. At about 2.30 or 2.45 I would generally become free. Then I used to make all the lacquer, after Lorenzo had shown me what to do. With alcohol, shellac and perfume I would make eau de cologne and setting lotion and he also showed me how to make permanent wave and how to dilute peroxide from a hundred-volume. It was very exciting to learn all these things. And then he realised quite quickly that I was very good at maths. I helped him doing some addition while he was doing the accounts and he said: 'My God, you're quick!'

'That's my forte,' I said. So I started to learn how to squeeze most out of a business not only by producing more income, but by keeping the costs down as low as possible. I was getting busier and busier. It was a very, very exciting part of my life working there: I was making a lot of money, I was extremely happy. I was starting to get an identity and learning a lot about business and about life. And I have something else to thank Mr Lorenzo for. Until I worked for him I was known by my real name, which is Giuseppe. My boss said firmly: 'Giuseppe is no good for hairdressing, we will call you Tony.' I changed that to Toni to make it look a little more Italian and I was perfectly happy with the change – I still am!

At that time I started doing about £50 or £60 and I even reached the magical £65 mark. You've got to think if I reached the £65 mark I was still taking home less than 30 per cent of that so Mr Lorenzo was doing very well out of me but I was extremely grateful to him for giving me such an opportunity. I was equally determined to move on to the next level. At 2.30 pm or so I would start again, doing the lacquer, then be back with clients at around 4.30 pm. Sometimes I would have six or seven clients. I had an assistant and I was assigned all those clients and I had to do them. They mostly came together and there would usually be one just for tinting so I would mix the tint for my assistant and she would put the tint on; I would do a perm while she did a shampoo. Then I would perhaps have to do a change of colour so I started putting the bleach on, then would do something else . . . I had to work very fast because I knew that by the end I had to finish all of the six or seven clients. It meant I could be at work until about 10 o'clock at night from 8 in the morning. I didn't mind the hard work because I was beginning to make really good money.

On a Saturday we finished at one o'clock. Then I looked at my turnover and usually I had surpassed the £65 mark. That meant anything I did after that would be shared equally with Lorenzo. Often we had Americans coming in, who liked us to use Coty lotion (it was like perfume with alcohol, which made the hair really shiny). We used to sell these for 5 shillings and 6 pence. We later learned that the alcohol would damage hair but at the time we didn't know this, otherwise we would never have done it. I was earning very good money. I would get £15 extra for staying, which meant £7 and 10 shillings for me. At that point my weekly total was reaching about £130 to £140, of which I would get about £60, plus some tips. It was a lot of money then, very good money. At the back of my mind there was the same thing spurring me on to earn more money so that I could buy my beloved mother her dream house. That was my greatest ambition.

THE CAPITAL OF THE WORLD

★　★　★

I would just like to flash forward for a moment to an occasion many years later when Lorenzo invited me to his house for lunch. He was in his early eighties by then and I was married with a young family. Lorenzo prepared a lovely three-course meal for us. I went with my wife, our four-year-old daughter and our son, who was three. It was amazing seeing him again, a very enjoyable experience. He then told me that in his fifty-year hairdressing career until I joined him he bought himself a flat, but in the two years that I worked for him he had been able to buy eight houses! This made me very proud. Mr Lorenzo became an inspiration to me. He never married but he had a nephew: Matthew Lorenzo, who became a well-known sports commentator on television. My old boss always talked about Matthew and was very proud of what his nephew had achieved; he was totally in awe of him. Years later I met Matthew Lorenzo Junior, who had followed in his father's footsteps and is today a sports commentator for Sky.

★　★　★

Returning to earlier days, before Lorenzo retired, my father left Renato's and Lorenzo said: 'If Toni is as good as this, his father must be even better!' So he asked me if I thought my father would like to come and work in the salon. I didn't mind at all. The idea of working with him again did not bother me now that I had a little more confidence. As I've said, my only aim was to earn as much money as I could and save it to buy my mother a house – that's all I was interested in. I was about eighteen or nineteen years old when I was working there, so I was growing up.

Little by little, I learned everything from Mr Lorenzo. He showed me how to do the PAYE, so I did all his wages and all the accounts every week. He showed me everything. It was quite a big salon and he used to sit at a higher desk at the back so that he could keep an eye on everyone. He was constantly telling people to hurry up and stop wasting time; he was keen to keep the clients happy.

I remember one time he was doing the hair of the Labour politician, Barbara Castle. Lorenzo was well over seventy years old and I could see that his shoulders were hurting as he lifted his arms to put the rollers in her hair. I said: 'I'll do it, Mr Lorenzo, it won't take me two minutes.' Although we were quite close he was instantly suspicious and said: 'I won't pay you any commission.' I said: 'Absolutely not,' so I stepped in and did it. As well as Barbara Castle, among the regulars was Mrs May, wife of the secretary of the then Prime Minister Sir Alec Douglas-Home. Mr May had also been secretary to several previous prime ministers, including Winston Churchill.

One day Mrs May invited me for tea and when I asked her for the address she told me 'at 10 Downing Street'. I couldn't believe it – I was dazed by the prospect of a young man from Scafati having tea at the home of the British Prime Minister. I caught a cab, but then I got so nervous about going into such an important house that I stopped the cab and panicked a little. I asked the cabbie to drop me off halfway, and I then walked the rest of the way. Arriving at Number 10, I was so terrified I didn't dare knock on the door. Eventually I plucked up the courage to do so and this giant policeman looked down at me and I was convinced I was going to be arrested. He said: 'Can I help you?' I said: 'Mrs May,' and he said: 'Oh yes, come in.'

Inside 10 Downing Street there was a little kiosk, which

the policeman went into in order to telephone Mrs May. She came to meet me and took me to her small apartment inside Number 10. We had tea together and a little chat. Her husband also very kindly asked me if I wanted to be shown around as the Prime Minister was away for the weekend. He showed me the Cabinet room and up the stairs there were lots of photographs of previous prime ministers taken from the early days. It was quite an experience for a young man from Italy already so much in awe of the British constitution.

My father worked on a commission-only basis at Lorenzo and while we started at eight o'clock in the morning he used to wander in at midday to Lorenzo's considerable consternation. My father did not really respect Lorenzo. In fact, he said he thought he was 'a crap hairdresser who just happened to have a shop'. To be honest, I think he was really a little bit jealous of him. So the two of them did not hit it off at all. That made life more than a little bit difficult for me because Lorenzo said he wanted me to become his partner. I said: 'What about Mr Paul, he has been with you a lot longer than me?' He said: 'Forget him, I want you to be my partner and I will give you 50 per cent of the business.'

At that time we paid £14 rent and the Conservatives had planned to redevelop all of Victoria Street so the salon was going to be knocked down, which meant we were on a rolling lease and the rent would not go up. Lorenzo was encouraging me to go in with him 50–50 and suggesting we could get another shop a little further down Victoria Street. He was going to invest all the money to set it up. I was very excited about this opportunity, but in the event, I moved on and a change of government stopped the developments, so Lorenzo remained in Victoria Street for many years to come at the same rent.

At that particular time I went from strength to strength in the business because all the clients wanted to go blonde. Unfortunately, with the techniques of the time, once you had bleached hair it turned a yellow blonde. There was nothing on the market at the time to make a proper Swedish blonde. But with the help of my father, we devised something special. Everybody had bleached yellow hair. We took a dye from L'Oréal Imedia 9.1, which was a very light ash blonde. I would squeeze four or five inches into a bowl and mix it with 20-volume peroxide to make it quite liquid and with a little bit of a thick conditioner called miracle mix and a shampoo. After we bleached the client's hair it would still be quite yellow so we carefully applied the magical mix, which killed the yellow so we were able to change it to an almost platinum blonde.

Of course the clients were very excited by this. I suppose there were not many places offering such a treatment – in fact you could say I was the first one to concoct the first platinum tint and maybe the first cream peroxide. As they did not exist until then when the news got round of course I became busier than ever, with all the directors' wives who wanted to become blondes. Until I started no one could become a platinum blonde, suddenly they all could, so that was a tremendous achievement. (Many years later I was feeling a little cocky and proud and I explained to L'Oréal that I had made up a platinum-blonde dye long before them.) And it really gave us the opportunity to cut costs. With my accounts head on, I saw how we could make a good business of it. At the time I was in heaven at the prospect of making enough money to buy my mother a house. Having 50 per cent of the business I thought I could very soon be financially secure.

The move to Clapham had given us somewhere better to live and with more money coming in and everyone in the family getting increasingly used to life in England, all seemed happier. My mother used to make wonderful meals of pasta, antipasti and meat and there always seemed to be friends around to join us at mealtimes. My father would go to Smithfield Market and buy half a cow. He used to get grapes from Covent Garden and we made our own wine in the garage. We had long, joyous family times with a few friends and neighbours to help us along. And lots of hairdressing went on at home as well: the kitchen was the starting point for the many visitors keen to have their hair styled.

My mother and father were very generous and hospitable. One of our frequent guests was Gino Annunziata, an old colleague and friend of my father's from Italy. He was a relation of Biagio. Gino was a devoted communist and a very good speaker; he often gave political party speeches in the piazzas, back in Italy. My father, being the kind-hearted person that he was, frequently invited him for lunch to our house. Gino had nine brothers and sisters, and was saving as much as he could, regularly sending money to Italy to help his family. He was very 'careful' with his cash.

The first time Gino was delighted and very complimentary. He told her 'what a fantastic meal' and then he explained to her that he was on his own and he had no friends in England, so my mother told him to come to our house whenever he liked. There were seven of us but she said: 'One more, one less makes no difference, so please come.'

After that Gino would be there every Sunday, regular as clockwork but always arriving empty-handed. Even so, we still always had a lovely typical Italian meal prepared by my mother. There was a sort of routine in those days when before lunch we used to go to the pub. While my mother was getting the meal ready, my father would take us for a drink. He would buy everyone a drink, including Gino. He'd say: 'Thank you very much.' And he'd say the same to a second one. Every week this happened until I had had enough and I said to my dad: 'It seems a bit odd this guy comes every Sunday without bringing anything. He eats and fills up to the maximum of himself, and he gets a drink before. It would be nice if for once he offered to buy you a drink, Pop.' My father said: 'Oh, it doesn't matter,' but he must have thought about it because the next time we went to the pub he bought the first round and then when it came to the second, he said very respectfully: 'Ah, Signor Gino, it would be very nice if you buy the second round.'

There was silence, and then Gino said: 'How can you think about another drink when your poor wife is working hard, preparing all the food for us and we are enjoying ourselves? Come on, let us go and help her.' It made my father look like an idiot and Gino still didn't buy a drink!

This happened early on in our time in England and there were many more wonderful meals for family and friends, including Gino, with whom I found myself having many profound discussions. In spite of his meanness I started to enjoy his company. To me he was like an open encyclopaedia; a man with a lot of life experience, he seemed to know many interesting things about life in general, and being a politician made him very persuasive with his ideas. I also learned a lot about cooking from him. He was very clever in utilising whatever ingredients were around to make a delicious meal in an extremely economical way. In fact, he was very economical full stop and everything he did got him a long way with very little to begin with. These important lessons later became the education and a base to create a profitable business for my company.

Politically, I never saw eye to eye with Gino, as he was a devoted communist, but I was surprised when this little guy was one of the first to have the courage to go and visit the USSR. He flew to Moscow at the time of Khrushchev and the Cold War and the visit made a huge impact on him. After he experienced the grim reality of a week in Moscow he returned very disillusioned by the experience so he then became a socialist, which pleased me no end! I certainly admired his courage and his conviction even though I never admired his tightfistedness. All the same, he has become a special family friend, whom I have known since I was fourteen.

It was always my mother who held the family together. She was wonderful in every way, but there was a secret sadness about her. More than anything on earth she wanted to have a daughter. The desperate need she had to give birth to a baby girl was always with her. Looking back, I can almost feel her pain. My mother was brave and beautiful, but she was not a strong person and her health was always terrifyingly fragile. I could not produce a baby daughter for her, but I kept alive my ambition to buy my mother a house, and this drove me on to earn as much money as I could. But I was soon to learn a cruel lesson that not all of our dreams come true.

CHAPTER THREE

A TURNING POINT: THE FIRST TONI & GUY SALONS

They say that if you can remember the 1960s you weren't there, but I can remember many things: from the line-up of the great Double-winning Spurs team I used to watch to the installation of John F. Kennedy as the youngest-ever President of the United States. I can recall the Berlin Wall going up, Yuri Gagarin blasting into space and the Beatles bursting on to the music scene. They were exciting times, and not just because I was young.

As sixties London famously began to swing into vibrant life it seemed on the surface that everything was really improving for the Mascolo family. Our home in Clapham was a much happier place than the cold basement in Islington where we had begun our time in England. The money I was earning had opened my eyes a little to the potential of hairdressing as a career. With his characteristic charisma my father had established a string of excellent clients to keep him busy and my brother Guy was doing very well in the family profession in a salon called Paulette in Clapham Park Road, not far from our home.

The only dark cloud in the blue sky of the family's future was the ailing health of my mother. She had only one kidney and she was becoming increasingly frail. The long years she had spent caring so devotedly for us all were really beginning to take their toll. Not only that, although she was fiercely proud of her five sons, her deep desire for a daughter really seemed to get her down. I know she had been extremely troubled by the loss of her first-born little girl. She also had several miscarriages, which must have distressed her greatly.

During our time in England she had to make a great many visits to the doctor and the hospital. Very often my father was busy working or away somewhere and I would be the one who would take my mother to most of her appointments. I never minded this task for I adored her very deeply, as you will perhaps have gathered by now, and besides it meant I got to spend more time with her.

At the suggestion of the wise Mr Lorenzo, I had grown a moustache to make myself look older (he thought it would make me more acceptable to clients and I happily agreed). But as my mother was always very slim, attractive and young-looking this also had the strange effect of leading people to believe she was not my mother, but my wife! Many times I had to correct nurses or receptionists and point out that we were not, in fact, a married couple but mother and son.

My mother never mastered English so I also had the role of translator, which meant I heard her medical problems first hand. This only served to increase my concern for her, especially when she had a consultation with a doctor when she again became pregnant. The doctor spoke no Italian so he had to explain to me that I must give my mother the awful news that if she went ahead and had the baby she was carrying, then it would almost certainly mean losing her own life. He spelled it out very carefully for me: 'If she has this baby then she will die for sure. We can take the baby away and she will survive, but it is not our decision. It has got to be her decision. If she wants to go ahead and have the baby, we will try our best but I can tell you the chances of her surviving will be almost nil.'

With a very heavy heart I translated this grim diagnosis to my poor mother, and asked what she wanted to do. With a selflessness that was so typical of her she replied: 'There is no question about it – I have lived forty-three years, the baby has not lived at all yet. It has to have a chance of life. I've already had my life.'

Shattered by her decision, I instantly decided to reverse it. I could not face the future without my mother so I ignored what she had said to me and told the doctor to abort the baby. I said: 'If you can save my mother's life and it means getting rid of the baby, then do it.' It might seem a dreadful decision on my part but to me at the time it was simply the right thing to do.

After that ordeal my mother went to Italy for a while, but her health never really improved. She was a very innocent and trusting person who believed just about anything anybody said to her. She was brought up to think the best of people and we would often hear her say: 'He would not lie,' if we questioned what someone had told her. Back in Italy she had visited some fortune-tellers, who had warned her to be very careful in all future medical matters. They said that if she had another operation she would surely die and she believed what they had told her was most certainly the truth. Then later, she developed a stone in her gall bladder. Her medic, Dr Smith, tried to reassure her that the operation needed to remove it was a very simple one but my mother was extremely concerned about the prediction. She understood perfectly well that it was a simple operation but she still did not want to let it go ahead because of the fortune-tellers.

It was a terrible time and I became increasingly worried. She lost a lot of weight and grew thinner and thinner. My father was away again and my poor mother was close to collapse when she was finally rushed to London's Italian Hospital on Dr Smith's instruction. He said everything would be fine and that there was really nothing to worry about but I still had a deep-seated feeling of unease. She had the operation and when I arrived at the hospital I was greatly relieved to hear Dr Smith say that everything had gone perfectly to plan. In fact he said it had gone: 'Fantastically well.' But when I went to her room and saw her, I instantly knew differently: it was plain that my poor mother was in a very bad way. As soon as I went through the door my heart sank. I was struck by a terrible feeling of shock and horror that I never want to experience again. My mother looked like a shadow of herself. She was so weak, she could hardly speak and she seemed as if she could never survive. She was like someone with no life left in her. I don't know if they could have saved her by giving her a blood transfusion or something. I remember sitting by her bed with a dreadful sinking feeling that she was slipping away. The doctor reassured me afterwards that she would recover and be all right but I think we both knew even then that this was simply a forlorn hope. It was awful, I never want to feel like that again.

On 12 December 1962 my mother died and my whole world felt as if it had been smashed apart. I couldn't understand why God had made it happen. It was so wrong that she died. At the age of just forty-five the life of my beautiful, radiant, loving mother ended far,

far too soon. 'Her heart gave up,' said the doctor. 'It wasn't strong enough.' It was absolutely the worst thing in the world that could have happened as far as I was concerned. For a time I felt suicidal. When I saw her lying in the mortuary she looked so young, just like a twenty-year-old, and at peace at last. Her complexion was beautiful and she had no lines on her face. I still feel her loss as strongly, half a century later; she is always in my mind and I know she always will be. She was a wonderful woman.

The loss of my mother hit me very, very hard, but of course it was traumatic for all of the family. She was the heart and soul of the Mascolo household and without her we were left lost and reeling. It felt as if our whole world had collapsed. I think we all turned into different people because of my mother's death. Probably my youngest brother Anthony suffered the most because he had such a short time with her, but we would all have been much better human beings had my mother lived longer. My father went to pieces and my younger brothers were all devastated. I was twenty when she died while Guy was eighteen, and Bruno was fourteen. Poor Andrea was just nine and Anthony was only five years old. It was perhaps hardest on the youngest two as we decided they should go to boarding school. Of course it was a tough decision to make but it was the only way we felt we could cope. They went to Copthorne Preparatory School in West Sussex, and although it was for the best, they hated being away from home.

★　★　★

It was left to me to try to pull the family together. Although totally consumed by my own grief, somehow focusing all my efforts on keeping things going helped me through the agony of our terrible loss. If we had been back in Italy then a large extended family would have helped us, but my dad and my brothers were all the family around. I knew it was down to me to take responsibility for our future. It was what my mother would have wanted, so all thoughts of travelling or any other sort of career were forgotten.

My job at Lorenzo's was the first thing to go. At first it seemed to me that the healthy income I was then earning would be needed by the family but I quickly realised, if I did not know it before, that there are things that are much more important in life than money. My father believed that Lorenzo was taking advantage of me and advised me to leave. It was decided I should try to come and work closer to our home in Clapham. Guy had left Paulette about six months earlier and was working at a salon just down Clapham Park Road called Cecil's, which was run by a Mr Cecil Moss. My dad said: 'Maybe Guy's boss could give you a job.' But it turned out that Mr Moss wanted to sell us the business.

★   ★   ★

Everything happened very quickly, and at a time when we were all, frankly, still in shock. My father never liked to work for anybody else and I think he was probably thinking about himself rather than about me. I thought he was wrong at the time, but I knew I must do everything I could to support the family. It was a big, big responsibility for me. When I first met Guy's boss, Mr Cecil Moss, I was delighted to find he was a charming, kindly sort of man. He was also a keen musician, which is what he wanted to spend his time on rather than being a ladies' hairdresser. He was then in his late thirties and wanted to retire from regular work to concentrate on his music before he was 'too old' to forge a career in music. When we met he said straight away: 'Look, I want to retire.' He wanted us to take over the salon and he offered us a twenty-one-year lease including all fixtures and fittings, contents and equipment, lock, stock and barrel. He had it all worked out and suggested we could take over the business for £20 a week.

This offer was not nearly as generous as it might sound today. Compared with the stylish working conditions I had enjoyed in the West End, the salon was awful. There was dreadful yellow lino on the floor and the whole place looked run-down and tatty. At the end of 1962 I would estimate the proper commercial rent for a small place like Cecil's would have been £2 or £3 a week, so he was certainly not doing us any favours financially. He had been left the whole building by his mother. The salon was only a small area at the front of the ground floor, with just a grubby little staff room and a toilet on the first floor. Upstairs there were flats, which were already rented out to people.

The salon might have been scruffy and run-down, but it was busy. Guy was the stylist and already he was very much in demand. There were some girls working there as well. It was making money, but it was a million miles from the elegant, upmarket salon of Mr Lorenzo, where clients paid a great deal more for their hair styling. I did not have much time to make up my mind, though: Christmas was fast approaching and I knew the family needed me so I decided, as the English saying goes, that 'beggars can't be choosers' and accepted Cecil's offer. The address of our brave new enterprise was 40 Clapham Park Road and my first business telephone number was MAC4275. I'll never forget it. As we opened for customers as the new proprietors I just hoped and prayed that the phone would keep ringing.

TONI: MY STORY

★   ★   ★

Toni & Guy started trading in January 1963, although the sign with our names on it did not go up until much later in the year — we were far too busy keeping the new business afloat in the early days to worry about that. Fortunately we were never short of clients. Guy was so good-looking and attractive to women that he was a great draw. In fact my father said we should just put a big picture of my handsome brother in the window and it would surely lure the ladies in!

In the first week we took a grand total of £72, which was a huge drop from the sort of money that was generated at Lorenzo's. And now each week I had to pay the £20 rent and all the bills and wages before Guy and I could have a penny. That first week I recall we were left with about £3 or £4 each plus a few tips. It was an enormous change for me. The rent was too much — you really can't run a successful business paying almost 30 per cent of your income in rent. The maximum should be 10 per cent. One minute I was earning £30 or £40 a week with no one to worry about but myself, the next I was barely scraping a living, with the responsibility for the whole family on my shoulders. It seemed impossible.

Like rats in a corner, we had no alternative but to make a success of it so we worked incredibly hard. We had no choice, we had to make it work. The first thing I did was to get the money to pay the rent, then pay the girls, pay the electricity and all the other costs. Whatever was left was what the family had to live on. We mostly lived on tips — it was enough to keep going but only just. Fortunately the rent on the house was only £5.

We just managed to make it pay because we worked very, very

hard. I did all the accounts and worked out all the money (Guy was not the least bit interested in that aspect of the business). And I did everything I could to keep our costs down. I even acquired a magnet so that I could go round on my hands and knees picking up all the pins from the floor. Normal practice in salons is to simply sweep them up and open a new box the next day, but I wanted to save every possible penny. I put the pins in boiling water with disinfectant and re-used them. Having learned all the techniques at Lorenzo's, I also used to make our own setting lotion and hair lacquer. I did anything I could think of to save money. We were determined to attract as many customers as possible and so we had thousands of leaflets printed advertising Italian hairdressing at its best with 'Florentine elegance, Venetian style and Roman flair'. It hardly seemed to matter that we hadn't been to any of those Italian cities! We walked miles round the streets of Clapham and the surrounding areas pushing our first advertising campaign through every letterbox we could find.

Gradually more and more clients came but we quickly found ourselves with an acute staffing problem. Soon after we took over, almost all the girls, both the young part-timers and the Saturday girls, decided to leave. I hadn't altered their wages or their conditions of employment, but it seemed in those politically incorrect times that they simply 'Didn't want to work with bloody Eyeties,' as we were described in those days.

To be honest, I know that many people who take over already-operating businesses find the existing staff choose to move on quite swiftly but also I must accept that I was perhaps not the easiest person to work for at this time. I was told that the girls thought I was arrogant and unfriendly. The truth is that I was not really arrogant, I was just very, very worried about the business.

And the death of my mother was still very raw and painful. I did not take the departing girls' attitude as racist, though I suppose in all honesty that is what it was; I just thought it was a very odd way for them to react. I never felt inferior. I think really they left because they felt I was too bossy with them and I was sorry because I liked them. I would have liked to have been friends with them and worked with them. Although I didn't take it personally, it did make life more difficult for me for a while.

There was just one English girl who did not abandon us at this difficult time, a rather pretty fifteen-year-old called Pauline. I first met her just a few days after my mother died and thought to myself how cheerful and attractive she was. Although romance was a million miles from my thoughts at that time, I remember thinking how much I liked Pauline as soon as I saw her. In fact I think I fell in love with her with all my heart from the very moment I first saw her. Perhaps deep down inside somehow I even knew that she was the woman I would one day marry. But in any case there was a problem: she was already going out with my brother Guy so I had to keep my feelings to myself for a while. I did get to see quite a lot of Pauline – at work of course but also because as well as working in the salon, she used to came to our house and help out an awful lot. I soon learned she was very kind and thoughtful, as well as pretty.

Pauline recalls:

The first time I met Toni Mascolo he frightened me half to death. I was working in the shop with Guy. I was cleaning, which is one of the jobs I've always loved to do, when I suddenly saw this person peering in the window. It was dark outside and he scared me. I turned to Guy and said: 'There's someone looking in the window.' Guy just said: 'That's my brother.' I was introduced and was shocked at first at how different the brothers seemed, though after a while I realised there were lots of similarities.

It was just so sad them losing their mother and I could see it was a terrible time for them. I was going out with Guy, but it wasn't a serious relationship. He was very good-looking and he liked to go out with lots of girls. I was very young and Guy and Toni were two of the first men from outside my family that I had ever properly encountered. I went to an all-girls' school and I never went out to clubs or parties, or anything like that. My father was Irish and a strong Catholic. The Church meant a lot to him. In those days you never went out with someone that you were not intending to marry – they were very different times from today. My parents really liked Guy at first, but we were just kids going out together as friends. It wasn't a big romance.

When the brothers took over the shop it was a huge surprise to all the staff. There were about six girls employed because in those days there weren't many boys who went into hairdressing. Most of the girls said straight away that they were not going to work for Italians – that's what life was like back then. They were very different days. I was the only one who stayed on. I think I felt so sad for them that I wanted to help them all I could.

I was only fifteen but after a while I used to go to their house when I wasn't working and clean the place and help to do the cooking with their dad. I just loved them so much, especially the two little ones, Andrea and Anthony. I always looked after Anthony as much as I could as he was just a baby; even to this day I love him so much as I love all of my family. I used to stay round at their house until 10 o'clock at night doing jobs and helping out. I would do anything if I thought it would make them feel happy. Although there was obviously a lot of sadness for them, there was also a lot of happiness for me. It was a really magical time. When they took the salon on it was very hard for them. Things were tough for Guy and Toni and they had the little ones to look after as well as the business.

Guy was always more relaxed and easy-going while Toni simply never smiled. I found that really sad. He just did his clients' hair and then spent the evenings either doing the books or working late in the salon. He soon started making his own lacquer and other things and sometimes I would help him. He was just so totally focused on his desire to make more money to provide a better living for the family. He never, ever thought about himself. I can't remember a single moment when he sat down and thought about what he wanted. He was always solely concerned with what he needed to do for the family.

Toni was totally different to Guy and their father. The dad was a lovely, lovely man, but like Guy he was a big show-off. He would come into the salon every day, looking immaculate in a smart suit with a carnation in his buttonhole. He was good-looking like Guy and they both loved life and they both loved women. They never seemed to worry about the family's financial position, they just thought they could do some more haircuts and make some more money. So it was left to Toni to do all the worrying. He was the one who felt he had to take charge of things. Toni automatically steps into that role – he always feels he has to look after everyone and be responsible. He's still the same to this day.

Looking back now, this was a time of great turmoil in all our lives. My mother's death really was the turning point for everything. It was strange that I should meet Pauline, who was to play such an important part in my life, so soon after she died. And it took me some time to realise that they are similar in many ways – they certainly both always made sure that everything was spotlessly clean. My mother used to make the floors so clean you could eat from them and Pauline is the same. But on a deeper level they both have great qualities of utmost reliability and decency alongside beauty that is much more than skin deep.

I soon found out that Pauline had spirit as well as looks. Early on in our time in Clapham, when I was still striving to keep our costs down, I saw her doing a tint and opening another tube when a tube was already opened. I asked her why she didn't finish the open tube, which was still half-full, and she responded by throwing it at me and saying, 'You do it yourself!'

I didn't say anything like that to her again as I could see she was working just as hard as Guy and myself to make a success of the salon. At first it was still known as Cecil's but after a few months my brother and I put our names above the shop and Toni & Guy was born. Fortunately, the clients seemed to like us a lot more than the staff did, and we were very busy from the start. Our customers loved to come to us because of the family atmosphere. They said that sometimes when they visited a more traditional hairdresser there was an atmosphere you could cut with a knife while coming to us was like being part of a family. Of course it was like that because we *were* a family: we worked for each other and we motivated each other. In those early days we founded the philosophy of Toni & Guy, which is to work as a team that is also a family. Whatever we had, we shared.

My share seemed to include doing most of the practical tasks and all the book-keeping. Guy was a hugely talented and very artistic hairdresser but he was not so good at some of the other necessary jobs. If I left him to answer the phone it would ring forever. I hated to see the place look untidy so it was always me who swept up. If I asked Guy to clean the floor, he wouldn't see that it needed doing properly. So I did all those jobs. There would be people waiting and Guy wouldn't notice because he always assumed 'Toni will do it'. I couldn't bear to see a mess on the floor or to find there were people waiting so I would deal with that. But he could be much more alert if there was a pretty girl around. If he saw I had someone attractive booked in, he would often ask her: 'Who's doing your hair?' and if the answer was Toni, he would quickly add: 'Well, he's quite busy. You don't mind if I do her, do you, Toni?' And of course I had to say: 'No, that's fine!' But we still had a lot of fun working together.

Our father was not around so much at the start of us running the Clapham salon. He had been very much in love with my mother and her death completely shattered him. Guy and I started the business in the depths of winter. The Big Freeze of 1963 – for the UK one of the coldest winters on record. Snow was left in the streets of Clapham for many days that seemed forever, it was bitterly cold. It was later on in the spring when my father came in and said: 'Oh, I'll help you as well.' In the summer he suggested that we form a company, and so F. Mascolo and Sons Ltd came into being on 31 August 1963. We split the business 33 per cent each to me and to Guy, with my father having 34 per cent. Before that we were 50–50, but the important thing was it was still a family affair.

★ ★ ★

Pauline was remarkable. She used to come to this house with five Mascolo brothers in it, with my father there were six men, and she just wanted to help. She learned the Italian way of cooking, with its two or three hundred years of recipes, so she could cook for us and she would help to clean the house. She was only fifteen, just a child really, but she was so keen to roll up her sleeves and do anything she could to help. Pauline's parents were really angry with us for a time. They said to her: 'Why are you working so hard for those Italians? What are you doing there all the time?' She said: 'I am really happy, I just want to help.'

She was not the type of girl who liked to go out dancing all the time. Quiet and shy, she didn't seem to have a lot of self-confidence. Other teenage girls would have probably been partying or going out with their friends clubbing but she was quite happy to stay in and be mumsy and look after us. She was really pretty and she did her hair up beautifully. I think she liked the warmth and liveliness of our place.

★ ★ ★

In November that year of 1963 the American President, John F. Kennedy, was killed. They say everyone old enough can remember where they were when they heard the news. I certainly can. I was styling the hair of my last client of the night, a nice lady called Mrs Price. I recall she had arrived at 8.30 pm, which serves to remind me of just how hard I used to work in those days. My brother Guy had gone out to the cinema with Pauline. I had the radio on in the salon and when the news came through both Mrs Price and I were deeply shocked. Already I was living with a permanent hurt from the loss of my mother but the assassination of the young American leader upset me deeply. He seemed such a young and inspirational figure and the United States was like the land of the future so when he was so savagely shot dead it was an enormous shock. I know I was totally devastated. To me John Kennedy embodied so much hope and goodwill in a troubled world that his death was a real blow; it was terrible.

The first year was very hard. We were still grieving yet we had to work as hard as we could all the time. The biggest problem came as 1963 ended and 1964 began. We had just established ourselves in a year of great effort and then came another bad winter. Big snowfalls stayed around for about a month, even in Clapham in London. It was a cold, horrible time and of course the effect on our business was horrendous but we still went in and worked six days a week. We would open up early on Monday and work solidly all the way through until Saturday night. It was very depressing and very cold. Obviously it was harder for some of our clients to come and have their hair done but we still worked hard to bring in as much money as we could.

At times like this you need all the good cheer you can get and often I found it came from my clients. Many of my regular customers became friends and one of my favourites was a little old lady who was well into her seventies. I loved doing her hair because she was very interesting and intelligent and she always liked chatting. Even in those days everyone seemed afraid of getting old, but this lady was so full of life and laughter and always looked so nice in her crisp white blouses that I never thought about her age. I remember in the depths of the worst weather I was doing her hair when a fairly wretched-looking older woman walked past the window. She looked very miserable and sorry for herself and an expression of concern must have gone across my face but my client smiled and said: 'Toni, don't worry. She was like that when she was eighteen! It's not age, it's attitude.' And that was a great lesson to me. She was a like a little ray of sunshine to me at that very grim time.

Sometimes I thought of Lorenzo and his elegant salon and the good money I could have been earning, but I tried not to dwell on the past. The memory of my poor mother still dominated my thoughts and for the family I knew I had no alternative but to keep going. They were difficult times for all of us when the snow fell. The income from the salon was still small and the rent was high and sometimes it was hard to see any light at the end of the tunnel. Out of the misery there was only one thing that warmed my heart and that was the new friend I had acquired, a friend who was already very special to me. How many times in your life do you meet someone you know is really special for you, a real friend? That was Pauline. When I was often very low, which was often, she lifted my spirits. She was wonderful, even though we were only friends.

But nothing could be allowed to interfere with the business of hairdressing. Fortunately our hard work paid dividends because as the months went by we became busier and busier. Occasional customers often became regular clients as we always strived to give the best possible service. As summer followed spring we became increasingly busy. The salon was very small with hardly any reception or waiting area so we began to see ladies queuing outside on a Saturday to get their hair done. Just like Mitchell's, the greengrocer across the road, which was also very popular – usually on a Saturday afternoon there would be people queuing over there as well, to buy their vegetables for Sunday lunch. Clapham Park Road was a very ordinary street but somehow at that time we began to turn it into something special. Right from the earliest years there was a wonderfully friendly feeling to Toni & Guy. I loved the way our customers became our friends and enjoyed their visits to the hairdressers. Some of them would even see how busy we were and say: 'Can I make you a cup of tea? I know where everything is!' They would go off and make the tea while Guy and I used to laugh and say: 'Thank you very much.' This was customer service in reverse! We created a new type of hairdressing, it was like an excitement second to none. Now we wanted to go to the next level and have a chain of salons.

Although my father and brother were working alongside me as hairdressers they were both more than happy to leave all the accounts to me. They always preferred to go out and enjoy themselves rather than to bury their heads in the books. I think I knew that I needed someone to turn to for the occasional piece of help or advice. Again I was very fortunate, for this was the time when I found the man who was to become my trusted financial adviser in the shape of an insurance broker by the name of Jack Feak. We first met when the charismatic Mr Feak knocked on the door of the Clapham salon looking for business and we hit it off straight away.

Jack Feak had been a major in the British Army in the Second World War. He had served extensively in Italy and he spoke Italian beautifully. An imposing man with a confident, booming voice, he looked a little like a young Bruce Forsyth and he was certainly always upbeat and entertaining. He limped a little, thanks to a wartime injury, and he was a proper, military gentleman. Best of all he was totally honest and straightforward and he could do all sorts of important tasks from giving advice and arranging endowment policies to insuring everything from your house or car to your donkey! Jack Feak quickly became a very close friend of mine and many, many times afterwards I came to value his advice.

★ ★ ★

In the middle of 1964 I decided it was time for us to expand and take the first step towards my dream of a chain of salons. We took over another shop in nearby Streatham. It cost us about £2,000 to buy the business at 33 Leigham Court Road, where the telephone number I will always remember was STR 5663. My father went to work there and the Toni & Guy name went up over the shop. We were extremely busy in Clapham and I think perhaps we were at least partly trying to imitate the flamboyant businessman hairdresser 'Teasy-Weasy' Raymond, who was then in the well-publicised process of building up a large chain of successful salons. I chose Streatham because it was a more middle-class area than working-class Clapham and it seemed to me because it was a richer area there would be more money around to pay for top-quality hairdressing. But while our new customers might have lived in their own semi-detached or even detached houses, rather than in the council flats of Clapham, many of them were saddled with large mortgages so the tips were always better in Clapham.

One of the great bonuses of the Streatham salon was that our customers included many well-known Italian families, some of whom ran restaurants in the West End. So we met many people from our own country who were making their way in England just as we were, and many of them became good friends.

One other reason for opening a second salon was that the staff of our family business had an important addition in the shape of my brother Bruno. When he first left school Bruno decided against becoming a hairdresser – he wanted to build a business as a greengrocer instead. Perhaps there was something of the merchant in his blood from our mother's Gallo family. Anyway he made his choice and he was very definite about it. He used to have to get up early in the morning to go to Covent Garden in his little van to get all the fruit and vegetables. Often he would go with our friend David Small, who worked in the market and also lived in a top flat in Chelsham Road with his wife and two children. Bruno always liked someone with him – he loved to have company as it helped to give him lots of confidence. But it was not an easy way to make a living: selling the produce was difficult and it was one of many problems.

I think it did not take too long before Bruno noticed that while he was rising at the crack of dawn and lugging heavy bags around, we were starting work at 8.30 am and spending our days looking after clients, many of whom were attractive young girls! Not only that, we were making more money than him. Soon he decided to change careers and join us. He wanted proper training as, being a little big-headed, he wanted to be better than everybody else, and so we paid for him to go to the Morris Masterclass School of Hairdressing. Bruno arrived in the family business, bringing lots of modern ideas about styling with him. He had learned all the basic types of hairdressing that we probably had never learned ourselves – and a little bit about public relations too. Bruno was very, very ambitious and always inclined to want to jump more than one step at a time. With a second salon we had somewhere for him and so he went to work in Streatham with our father.

Soon after we opened our second salon the General Election in October 1964 ended thirteen years of Conservative rule and installed Mr Harold Wilson in Number 10, Downing Street. This was not good news for Great Britain but it turned into very good news for Toni & Guy, in my view.

While Harold Wilson's government was in power it was the worst of times in many ways. Inflation soared and the British attempt to join the Common Market was flatly rejected. Wilson dropped plans for the Channel Tunnel, changed the face of Rhodesia and dragged the country way down economically in the League of Nations. But the inflation he helped to cause really assisted our business because the crippling Clapham rent of £20 began to seem not such a drag on our business. We had the lease for twenty-one years so as time went on, it became an increasingly better deal. As it happens Wilson also cancelled the planned redevelopment of Victoria Street so Lorenzo's rent remained fixed for many years – meaning that I could have made myself a huge fortune there. No matter, that door was closed and Toni & Guy ended 1964 on a massive high.

★   ★   ★

Those first two years were hectic and for me, very much over-shadowed by the death of our mother. We all used to go to visit the cemetery every Sunday and I believe I was ill with grief for a long time. Perhaps that was why I focused on work so strongly. The clients kept coming and I found that completely losing myself in my work meant that my pain eased a little.

Our busiest-ever day in Clapham was Christmas Eve 1964. Everyone seemed to want their hair to look good for Christmas and we had so many customers we started early in the morning and finished at 10 o'clock at night. We treated the day as a show and it was amazing from start to finish. Guy looked after no fewer than sixty-four clients and I did fifty-nine. He was a bit quicker than me, and a better hairdresser; he was also more artistic. The girls brought in flasks of coffee and tea and sandwiches that their parents had made. It was a wonderful atmosphere. We all knew we had to pull out the stops to look after all the clients we had booked.

That day Pauline really came up trumps. She was always very, very good with long hair, excellent at all the beehives and curls that were popular in the sixties. In fact she had such an eye for it she did about thirty clients that day. At 8.30 pm I was exhausted and went into the toilet – the only place where you could get a bit of privacy – and closed my eyes for five minutes. Then I came out awake and refreshed. After we had finished we moved all the chairs and had some drinks and relaxed with an impromptu party. Some of the clients joined us and it turned into a very happy occasion.

It was quite an exceptional day. We were totally exhausted by the end, but very happy. I think we knew we had created something special.

CHAPTER FOUR

GOING
UNISEX

There are many aspects of the Toni & Guy story that give me pride and satisfaction. I believe there are lots of different ways in which we have helped to change and influence hairdressing all over the world, but perhaps our first major achievement was to create the unisex salon. In London in the 1960s, like most places in the world, women went to hairdressing salons while men went to barber's shops, and they remained traditionally very different establishments. But in 1965, in Streatham, we established one of the world's first unisex salons. Like a great many good business ideas, it began life in direct response to requests from our customers. As the Streatham salon found its feet my father and my brother Bruno kept reporting that a lot of ladies were inquiring: 'Can you cut my husband's hair?' or 'Can you cut my son's hair?' And the same questions had already been asked of Guy and me in Clapham many times before.

It was at a time when everyone was becoming increasingly

fashion-conscious and aware of their appearance and obviously there were lots of men who hankered after something more than the old short back and sides. The demand was there so we thought, why not? We welcomed the menfolk of our female clients and quite soon we had a good number of male customers and turned it into a proper unisex salon. In fact I think we were the first unisex hairdressing salon in the world.

Bruno had brought a lot of new ideas to the business and soon our youngest brother Anthony was also knocking on the door. He was only twelve when he first joined the fraternal hairdressing line-up. It was a very busy time at Clapham and I asked one of my assistants to look after the next client. 'Oh, no!' was the horrified response. 'She shouts and she is difficult.' I said: 'Look, I'm busy, I can't do everything.' Schoolboy Anthony just happened to be in the salon at the time and he jumped in and shouted: 'I'll do it, I'll do it!' And sure enough he did it. From an early age he was brimming with great confidence: he would chop people's hair with enormous spirit, he had no fear at all. My father pushed him the same way he had pushed me. He would say: 'You have watched me for long enough, you do it.' Soon Anthony was doing it very well indeed. My father's attitude helped to give him the courage and strength to do it.

In many ways my father was a remarkable man and he never lost the ability to surprise me. Quite a while after my mother had died we asked him if we could have a party at the house and invite some girls round. My father said it was OK by him, so long as we invited one for him! I thought he hadn't got a chance with all the young girls we knew but he was only in his late forties, always a charmer and very smartly dressed. He knew how to talk to the girls and in that first party, and in quite a few parties afterwards, he seemed to hit the jackpot. We were very surprised and very jealous too.

I was never as successful with the opposite sex as my father and brothers but I did have my moments. I once went out with a very pretty girl called Carol while Guy was seeing her friend Jennifer. I thought both girls were very feminine and pleasant, but I got a shock when they clashed with two other girls who were on the other side of the street. Suddenly out of nothing a huge row broke out between the girls. There were screams and shouts and I could not believe my eyes when Jennifer punched one of the other girls. I said: 'What did you do that for?' Jennifer said: 'I don't like her and they were staring at us.' I discovered that while 'teddy boys' were a young people's movement I knew about, Carol and Jennifer considered themselves to be 'teddy girls'. I thought, *Wow, I'm going out with a 'teddy girl' – how exciting!*

We were all on a very steep learning curve in those days, me included. You had to be inventive at all times dealing with customers, especially those who wanted their second perm, because when they returned three months later their hair was no longer in a virgin state. If you used the same size curls and original setting lotion you would end up with different results therefore you had to be very inventive and astute and use a weaker lotion, maybe larger curls. You could say it was quite a challenge! No one ever taught me things like that – I had to find out for myself as I went along. Some ladies came in with totally bleached hair. If you touched it too hard, it would break. And they wanted a perm? A perm on hair like that could kill it and the tints and perms of today simply did not exist. You had to improvise with a few drops of ammonia in a little water with some conditioner, which would then be swiftly neutralised with peroxide to make sure the curls were like the original style. Talk about learning on your feet!

With the two salons running successfully I was determined to keep expanding and open a third. Already I had decided to employ Mr Paul, with whom I had worked at Lorenzo's. I found a place in Mitcham and it cost about £3,000 to do it up. I did it mainly to help out Mr Paul – he was my friend and a very good hairdresser and he needed a job. Pauline went there to work with him.

When I was out for the night at places like the Locarno, a dance hall in Streatham, I loved to tell everyone that I had three salons. To be honest I was not so interested in the money, it was the image of having three salons. I used to think it would impress the girls but I'm not sure it worked. I had a good friend called Arno who was much better than me at attracting the opposite sex: he was a good musician and he played the guitar at La Dolce Vita, which was *the* place to be seen in Soho. Arno always had girls eating out of his hand.

I had another business idea to use his musical and romantic talents: to get together and open a nice coffee bar in Chelsea. Of course this was in the days before they had been properly invented. Not for the only point in my life was I ahead of my time, but unfortunately Arno was not in the least bit interested. I used to meet him and we would go to the Empire, Leicester Square or the Locarno together. I thought he was amazing because he was so cool and relaxed; he would just wander round and talk to all the girls. I wanted so much to be like him but I was shy and not very confident.

Mind you, Arno was not so cool on one particular night when I met him in Café des Artistes. He was chasing after a stunning blonde girl who eventually agreed to let him walk her home. I was very jealous and thought he had really hit the jackpot. He left with a huge grin on his face but when I met him the next day he was absolutely mortified. It turned out he had gone back to her place and after he made a passionate pass he discovered that she was not really a girl at all but a boy! This was a very different time and things like this just didn't happen so you can imagine his shock.

With the accounts from three salons to keep on top of I was busier than ever, but I still found time to buy a convertible Triumph Herald, which was my dream car. Pauline really liked soft-top cars and I played a joke on her with it. I parked it near the salon in Clapham and said to her: 'I would love a car like that.' And she said: 'One day you'll have one.' Then I said: 'Let's go for a ride,' and I got in the car and said to Pauline that we could just go for a spin and then bring it back. She was very worried and thought I'd turned into a car thief. I said I was sure that the owner wouldn't mind and she began to get really concerned. She screamed that the police would arrest me, before I let on that I had already bought it!

I enjoyed joking with Pauline. She was not at all like the other girls. I saw a lot of her as she used to come and help us all out at home – she liked to be busy at our house and I loved to see her there. She was my best friend and at that time I daren't even dream of anything more.

Pauline explains:

I was like part of the family – all the brothers had made me like their little sister. I was looking after them and they were looking after me. Anthony was only little and he treated me like his mum. I really loved going round to help out at their home. They definitely needed a woman's touch but they were always so wonderfully warm and welcoming. I looked after them and they looked after me.

Then Guy went down with typhoid – that was another tremendous shock for the family. He was taken to hospital and we were all extremely worried because he was very ill. The salon was still really busy and I missed Guy's help, influence and support immensely but at least Pauline was still there helping me. She was my assistant back then and I adopted the technique of my father and pushed her on the floor to style and cut. I have to say she was a godsend. She quickly gained a lot of confidence and never looked back, just like me when my dad threw me in at the deep end.

Mrs May, my client from Downing Street, followed me from Victoria Street to the salon in Clapham even though it was a long distance out of her way. I loved looking after her – she was a wonderful lady who was always very kind and appreciative. And once again she invited me to tea. However, this time she also invited Pauline as she was helping me at the time. Mrs May became very fond of Pauline, and came to think very highly of her. So again I set off for Number 10, Downing Street for tea. I was less nervous this time round but still very worried. Pauline, bless her, was terrified; but nevertheless it was a great experience in our lives, a truly magical occasion for two young kids. Later, I was invited to go and see Mrs May again but this time she was in Albert House, a much more grandiose residence that was the Prime Minister's temporary residence when Number 10, Downing Street was closed for renovation.

Guy's illness was a great worry for all of us. For a time he was not at all well in hospital and Pauline wanted to visit and so did I. Naturally very often we went together. I think it was at that time that we became even closer, though I still kept quiet about my feelings for her. I was very honourable and never made any romantic moves. Certainly I never made a pass at her or anything like that. Gradually Guy recovered and came home from hospital but soon afterwards his relationship with Pauline ended altogether.

Pauline remembers:

Toni knew I was terribly upset when Guy became ill and he took me to see him many times. He was just as desperately worried as me; in fact he was beside himself when Guy contracted typhoid. Toni was still reeling from the death of his mother so it was hard for him when his oldest brother became ill. And of course there was much more pressure on him at the salon because there was much more for him to do. To be honest, I think I first fell in love with Toni at the time we were going to visit Guy but I never told him how I felt.

Fortunately, before too long, Guy got better. My relationship with Guy was over very soon after he recovered. It wasn't ever a big thing to either of us. After we broke up, I went to Italy for a while. I found myself a job looking after children, but as soon as I got there I wanted to be home with my family.

I was devastated when Pauline went away; I felt totally lost without her. I realised how much I relied on her and how much I cared for her. I had bought the shop and the business was going well; she was my best friend and she looked after us. There was no one else I wanted to be with. In actual fact I had fallen very, very much in love with her. I was extremely down and I thought no one else would really do for me: she was my dream girl. I just thought to myself that I would probably be depressed for a long time until somehow I got over it, or at least learned to live with it. I would never give up, but I was badly hurt inside. It was not as bad as when my mother died, but it was still very painful and I felt I had lost someone I loved very much. I knew then that she was the only woman for me. No one else would come close so although I'd always imagined having a wife and a family, I think I had resigned myself to living alone, concentrating on my work and taking care of the family.

Pauline recalls:

I hated being away from my twin sister Eileen and my parents more than anything. That was the worst thing. I missed my parents terribly but I think I missed Toni as well. I came back after about six weeks and straight away I phoned the Mascolos. Toni just said: 'We are all going out tonight. Why don't you come?'

I will always remember that night. I had a really soft spot for Pauline but I was still never sure if she really liked me or not. I was going dancing with a tall girl called Michaela, but she wasn't really my girlfriend. We went to the Empire, Leicester Square, and when we got inside somehow I lost Michaela so I said to Pauline: 'Let's have a dance.' When you start dancing you get close to your partner. I wasn't the best of dancers but I pretended I liked it – you can test if someone likes you when you're dancing. We danced together closely and I started to think that she really liked me. Already we knew each other quite well as friends. I suppose I was in love with her anyway but I didn't want to overdo it. There were obviously feelings between us but for a while we remained just good friends.

Pauline remembers the night:

My father was really funny and insisted I was home by 10 pm. Toni was going with his cousin and another girl. We went to the Empire, where I'd never been before. It was nice and then Toni started dancing with me and this other girl went off somewhere. That was it. I think we both knew then that we really liked each other but we were both very shy. Times were very different back then. I was always very concerned about my parents' feelings. Compared with the behaviour of young people today we were very innocent.

Then one night soon afterwards Pauline came to the house and Carol came as well. (I hadn't given Carol up because I still wasn't going out with Pauline at this stage. We had just enjoyed a night dancing together.) I was a bit naïve when it came to girls really and I was going to drive them both home. Carol lived in Clapham while Pauline lived further away in Camberwell. I dropped Carol off first, without really thinking of the significance of what I was doing. 'I'll see you soon, Carol. I'll give you a ring,' I said. Her reply shocked me. She said: '★★★★ off! I don't want to see you again.' I was a bit innocent – I didn't really mean anything by dropping her off first, but she clearly thought I was showing it was Pauline I wanted to be with.

I didn't really care about Carol. After the night at the Empire when we danced together I was 100 per cent happy that Pauline was the girl for me. I always felt the same way about her.

Pauline says:

From then we started seeing each other, but I felt I couldn't go back to work for them because it wouldn't have felt right. So I got a job as a hairdresser in the City and worked there for about a year. Toni came and picked me up one night and looked at the books and he was horrified at how little

I was earning. He wanted me to come back and work for them. I said: 'Let's leave it and see what happens between us.' He didn't say anything to me about getting married and I certainly didn't want to say anything to him. I thought that perhaps he wasn't really that interested in me so perhaps I'd go off and get a job somewhere else. I was thinking of working on a cruise ship as a hairdresser. I didn't really want to do it but I didn't want to be stuck in a relationship that was not going to go anywhere. So I told him I was going off and he looked distraught. But he still didn't say anything. I wondered what he really wanted.

Anyway, when push came to shove I told my mum I didn't really want to go away on the boat because deep down I knew I'd be just as unhappy as when I went to Italy, and I wouldn't be able to get back so quickly. Instead I went on a family holiday with my mum, dad and sister, to the Isle of Wight. Toni was so pleased when I told him I hadn't gone on the boat. He couldn't understand why I had considered it in the first place. I said that I just didn't know where we were going. Then he said: 'But I want you to marry me! I thought you knew that – I just forgot to tell you!' I said: 'Great.' That was it really, and from that time we worked together and started to build everything up with all the brothers. But Toni and Guy and I were together for a long time before the others came in.

I knew Pauline was the woman I loved and I was so happy when we were finally together. But my friend Mr Paul was not impressed by her slim and attractive figure. He advised me in all seriousness that she would not be a good wife for me because she was not big and strong. He gravely advised me that instead I should find myself a girl with strong muscles and broad shoulders who would be able to do lots of work. I couldn't believe what I was hearing. I said to him: 'I am not buying a horse!' To be fair to him, he soon changed his tune after he had worked for a while with Pauline in Mitcham. He found that, in spite of her slight frame, she was an excellent worker.

Pauline remembers:

Toni and I decided to get engaged. We saw a ring in Hatton Garden and Toni bought it for me. That was it! We didn't have a party or anything. But it wasn't easy for us. We were both worried because I had been out with Guy first and that was always in the background. It worried me and I know it worried Toni as well.

I was very, very happy when everything was clear and Pauline was my fiancée. We had been good friends for such a long time it seemed like a natural progression. In a way she was already part of the family, I suppose, but now I knew the two of us were going to be our own family I could not have been more pleased. I have very warm memories of us together at Chelsham Road. My mother had made the house look stunning with beautiful carpets and elegant curtains. I used to have a desk in my little room and on a Sunday I would sit there and do all my paperwork. Pauline would come and sit and watch me. There was no television in those days. She would just sit and be there with me – her presence was always a great comfort.

I was very pleased she was there. It helped to give me the confidence to keep on doing the work and earning the money. Then she wanted to learn to drive. I said: 'I'll teach you to drive,' and I put L plates on my car. She was very nervous to begin with and early on when we were in a queue of traffic, she bumped into the back of the car in front. I quickly said: 'Don't worry, don't worry! It's only a tiny bump and he hasn't even noticed.' I got her to relax and start again. I continued to teach her and eventually she passed her test and got her driving licence. She loved driving. I thought, *That is great: now she can borrow the car and drive herself home!*

★   ★   ★

There is a lot of psychology about hairdressing. The clients love to come and have their hair done because the whole experience can make them feel good. To do that successfully, you must not show any signs of pain or sadness. Although I worked as hard as I could through all this early period of running salons I have to admit that for much of the time deep down I was still depressed. It took me an awfully long time to come to terms with my mother's death. I lost a lot of my hair soon after she died, my eyesight deteriorated and I had to wear glasses. And a little later I had a great deal of trouble with my teeth so I had to keep going to the dentist.

I was haunted by the fear that I was going to lose all my teeth – I even used to dream about it. I continuously got infections around my teeth because I had the wrong bite. My dentist gave me penicillin for a long time but it did not solve the problem. Eventually I developed pyorrhoea – inflammation of the tissue round the teeth – so I went to see a specialist at King's College Hospital to get it sorted out because I was in pain all the time. His diagnosis was quick and shocking: he needed to cut the gums and reorganise my teeth. The business was so busy I decided to have it all done in one day. I went in at eight o'clock in the morning and he cut the gums and cleaned the teeth before stitching up the gums and putting plasters over to help stop the bleeding.

I was in agony but I had to go straight back to work because I had a long list of clients booked from one o'clock. It was like returning to work right after a major operation and I would have given anything to go home, but I couldn't. I thought, *If I go home who is going to give me the money?* My first clients were a very elegant regular and her daughter. They were among our most important customers and of course people don't want you to be in pain if you're going to help them to look beautiful. My client could see I was in distress but I said: 'Nothing, I've just had a little problem with my teeth, but I'm fine. Let's carry on.' The pain was excruciating all that afternoon and the next day and for several days after that but eventually it wore off and I recovered. I did not take any time off because I could not afford to. I had to do it otherwise I would have been sitting at home worrying about the salon losing money.

You couldn't really make a great deal of money with three salons the way we were operating. Our costs were too high, but we worked hard and didn't do too badly. I started saving a bit of money and sharing the costs 50–50 with my dad, I bought our first house. It was in nearby King's Avenue and we bought it from a police inspector for £3,500. It was a small cottage with a garage and a nice little garden at the back, a bit like a doll's house. We all lived there and Pauline would come and look after us all. Again, she would just sit and watch me do the books. I needed the security that she gave me. There was no stress; I felt safe because I had been able to pay everybody.

Pauline and I have so many wonderful shared memories from those early days. After I met her I never wanted to be with another woman. Pauline was very precious and important to me and at first it was not easy to persuade her parents to accept me. Her father was very Irish and with my Italian accent it was hard for us to understand each other. When we met we would both be turning to Pauline and asking: 'What did he say?' Usually it would end in laughter, which was good.

He was a very decent, down-to-earth man, a plumber who liked his Guinness, and Pauline's mother was well up in the union party. I would argue that capitalism was the better system. As I got to know Pauline's parents better, I grew to like and respect them very much. Meeting their daughter was the best thing that ever happened to me.

CHAPTER FIVE

A LUCKY MAN

I will never forget the moment I asked Pauline to marry me. She looked at me with great seriousness and said: 'I love you and I'll marry you, but on one important condition. If we are fortunate enough to have a family, my children will always come first, even before you.' I was so happy to hear this, because I felt exactly the same way and that has not changed at all in all the years that have passed since then.

I am a very lucky man. I don't feel any different today about Pauline than I did the first time I saw her. She has always been the only woman for me. You can talk about all the business empires you have created and the fortunes you have made, but in my own estimation my greatest achievement is finding someone I really love to share my life with. What Pauline and I have between us is true love and that is priceless.

Our wedding was a wonderful occasion, but at first it seemed our happiness was to be denied. We wanted to be married at the

Italian Church. It was beautiful and ceremonies often took place on Sundays, which was the only day the salons were closed. It was our dream to be married there. However, when we went, very respectfully, to ask for permission to be married there I was surprised and horrified by the response. We were told in no uncertain terms that because Pauline was not Italian they did not feel she was a strong enough Catholic to be married there. I was outraged. This was totally opposite to the truth because I knew that she was a much stronger Catholic than I would ever be.

Pauline recalls the disappointment:

It was very hard to take. There was an old priest at the Italian Church when we went to ask for permission. Toni started talking to him in Italian and I could understand the language well enough to get the message when the priest said, 'What do you want to get married here for? She is English and she is probably not even a Catholic.' That made me really angry. I thought, *How dare you? I am more of a Catholic than he is, even if I am not Italian.*

But Toni was brilliant. He said, 'I'm not having him talking to us like that.' I was upset because we really needed a Sunday service because of the business and I thought that was the only place that did them. Hardly anyone got married on a Sunday, back in those days. So I went to my priest at my regular church up East Hill in Wandsworth to ask for help. He was very kind. He said, 'Don't worry. Let's see what we can do.' He telephoned me later and said, 'How would you like to get married in St George's Cathedral in Southwark?' We were thrilled.

I had always dreamed of having this huge, lovely, big

wedding, all in white and all wonderful but in my wildest dreams I'd never imagined getting married in a cathedral. It was an enormous place and it helped to make me feel really special.

On the day of our wedding Pauline looked absolutely, fantastically beautiful, of course. Southwark Cathedral is near the Oval cricket ground and it was a fabulous occasion. We had around 150 people on 23 August 1970 and the sun shone for us. The only time it rained was when we were inside for the service. I was twenty-eight years old and Pauline was twenty-three. I was the happiest man in the world that day. We couldn't afford to go to a hotel for an expensive reception, but instead we had a brilliant family celebration in the hall next to the cathedral.

Pauline says:

We had no money in those days so we had to do everything on a shoestring. My aunt did all the cooking but it was still a sit-down, four-course meal. Our families had decorated the hall and made it look really nice. We even had the service conducted by a friendly priest from the Italian Church, who unfortunately had not been on duty when we went to visit! The day after the wedding we went to my mum's for lunch and then we left for Italy for our honeymoon.

I had actually arranged two weeks off so we could have a proper honeymoon and so we flew to Italy and went to a hotel in Sorrento, not far from where I was born. It is a beautiful coast and there was so much there I wanted to show Pauline and so many people I wanted to introduce to my new bride. I was overjoyed with happiness, but our honeymoon did not go quite as I had planned it.

The first problem I encountered almost as soon as we arrived at the hotel. In those days a lot of students, many of them local Italians, were recruited to work in the hotels. I overheard some of the boys and young men discussing which girls they fancied and making arrangements about who was going to chat up which of the female guests. I realised they were even discussing girls who had not yet arrived at the hotel. And then I saw some of them had taken a shine to Pauline and had started to talk to her in a very familiar way.

I am not normally a jealous man but I was newly married and very much in love. I got a little bit upset because I had travelled to Italy, my own country, with my new wife and I expected a little more respect. In the end as young men approached Pauline I lost my temper. I said: 'Are you ****ing stupid? Are you crazy? Do you think I am not good enough? Bugger off! I've just got married. Go and play around somewhere else.'

Unfortunately that was not the only setback on our honeymoon. After only two or three days Pauline started feeling very sick. I thought she must have eaten something that disagreed with her. For the rest of the holiday she wasn't well at all. We found out later that she was not ill but pregnant! I thought: *My God! I can't believe it. Even after waiting all these years we can't even have a proper honeymoon!*

Pauline remembers:

At first when I felt sick I thought it was the effects of the coach trip around all those hairpin bends with a long, terrifying sheer drop to the bottom. Toni's friend Gino lent us his car, which I thought might not be so frightening, but he didn't tell us the brakes didn't work very well! We went to visit Toni's relatives every day and every house we went in served coffee. Everyone in his family was so welcoming and they all wanted to meet me, but I drank so much coffee I even started to think that might be causing my sickness. When I got on the bus to go back to the airport I was so sick all the way there. When we finally returned to England I was convinced I had typhoid as my symptoms seemed a bit similar to Guy's when he caught the disease. I couldn't believe I had become pregnant straight away. I said to the doctor, 'Surely nobody falls pregnant this quickly?' He just looked at me and smiled and said, 'They do.'

I had a test and of course that was it, I was expecting a baby. It was strange. I felt too ill to be pregnant so I couldn't even feel properly happy. Some women are the picture of health when they are pregnant, but not me. I felt horrendous throughout. It was our first year of marriage and we should have been having a fantastic time together but instead I was so ill I went back to live with my mum for a while. I couldn't even walk from one chair to another without being sick. I couldn't go in a car. It was a nightmare.

It was awful for Pauline. She had an incredibly hard time and there was nothing I could do to stop her feeling so ill. We were very busy at the salons so I was working hard and I just kept hoping that all would be well once the baby was born. As the date neared I learned that our baby was due to be born on 6 May, my own birthday. I was delighted and looked forward to a memorable double celebration. But as the last days ticked away Pauline became more than ever anxious to make the house look immaculate. She started rushing round and working terribly hard to clean the place up for when she came back from Dulwich Hospital with the baby. Of course by doing that she accelerated the birth by two days to 4 May! I was extremely angry because I wanted it to happen on my birthday.

But I forgot all that when the baby came into the world. It was the most unbelievable experience of my life, for our baby was a little girl, the first girl to be born into the Mascolo family for a generation. My mother, who had always yearned for a daughter and sadly never produced one, would have been so happy for us. I thought of my mother a lot. Her maiden name was Gallo, which means 'cock' or 'rooster' in Italian. Then she changed to the Mascolo ('masculine, male'), making a masculine cock. But now we had a baby girl, which so delighted Pauline and myself and our whole family.

Pauline recalls:

Toni was absolutely over the moon that we'd had a little girl, although when she was born he first thought she was a little boy because he could see the cord! We were both delighted when we realised she was really a girl. He stood and cried, he was so excited.

I telephoned my father first and then I went on to phone just about everyone else I knew. I was so excited that my first child was a girl, and felt so much for my mother that I was overcome with emotion. Naturally I wanted to call my daughter Maria after my mother, but my wife decided to be awkward and said she felt it was too old-fashioned. Pauline liked the name Sacha more, so we settled on calling her Sacha Maria. I had always imagined we were having a boy so I was very shocked and so, so happy. Normally Italians would always like to have a son first, but I wanted a daughter more than anything else in my life. I was a very happy man.

Little Sacha Maria changed me as soon as she was born. She was such a tiny, precious little thing I became instantly concerned for her protection. Pauline was in hospital with the baby for a week, which was the custom then, and I was quite a good driver so I went to the hospital myself to pick them up. In those days we didn't have seat belts or baby seats and when I got behind the wheel of the Triumph Herald with my very important passenger at first I couldn't drive – I was paralysed with fear that we might bump into something and my fragile new daughter would be hurt. I was frightened that someone might suddenly stop in front of us and she could hit her head; she could even die. I was absolutely terrified. My entire outlook on life was instantly altered. I think perhaps I knew I was over-reacting but I could do nothing about it.

Eventually I plucked up courage to set off for home in King's Avenue and I drove at about ten miles an hour. The car was crawling along and I was shaking with fear. Pauline told me to get a move on – she felt no danger because she was holding the baby. I tried to be more rational but it was very difficult. I lost all confidence. After an age we did arrive home safely but for a long, long time the arrival of a baby daughter into my life completely altered my priorities. I was so worried that something dreadful might happen to little Sacha Maria, I was protective to the maximum.

It was a difficult time for the mother as well. Pauline recalls:

We had been in the house together since we got married but we weren't exactly prepared for the baby. Little by little we had done the place up, one room at a time. Toni would do the decorating and I would do the curtains, but when we brought Sacha home from the hospital I only had one chair to sit on – we did not have any money to buy any more furniture. Toni would not buy anything we would have to 'pay off' for. If we didn't have the money, we didn't buy it. That's how he was and he is still a bit like that today.

So we had a bed and the bedroom done and the kitchen was fine, but I really did only have the one chair to sit and nurse Sacha. It was a tough introduction to motherhood. Toni brought me home from hospital with the baby, left me at the door and said, 'Right, see you later,' and went back to work (there was no paternity leave in those days). Toni worked very hard as always and he didn't used to get home until 10 o'clock at night. It was quite daunting and very difficult but I always had my own family to help. My twin sister had had six children of her own by then and she still found time to come round a lot to help. I needed it because Sacha simply never stopped crying. She cried from morning to night. I had her all day and Toni helped at night, but it was still horrendous at times.

Life was very different then. Even though it was hard I just got on with looking after the baby and the rest of the family because Toni's younger brothers were living with us for some of the time. I was a mother to them all. Anthony still remembers me taking him to my mum's and I love them all. They are all very different and all lovely in their own ways. People used to say, 'How can you be around them? They shout at each other all the time, they never stop arguing.' They were very passionate and they did argue a lot but it was always soon forgotten. They love each other.

I put it all down to their Catholic upbringing, where there

is a lot of fear about what can happen if you do anything bad. That's how I was brought up as well. Catholicism is all based on the family and they all needed a mum and although I could never really be their mother I was a very nurturing person. I enjoyed trying to look after them all. It was hard but when I was in that little house with my baby and Toni's family I might have been completely exhausted most of the time but deep down inside I felt like the luckiest person on the planet.

Then, very quickly, I found out that I was pregnant again. I couldn't believe it, but I had no choice but to get on with it. We couldn't afford any help. It was tough on Toni as well because he was really busy at work and then he had to come home and help me. I think that was the toughest time in our lives but we were happy as well as tired.

Pauline is a wonderful wife and mother and she coped brilliantly in those early days. I loved Sacha more than I ever thought possible but she was not an easy baby. When we found out we were going to have another child so quickly it was quite a shock. It was at this time that Pauline showed me in no uncertain terms how family always comes first. I knew we needed more space because the King's Avenue house was quite small. I had an opportunity to buy a much bigger house, with six floors, in Chelsham Road, near where we used to live, for £22,000. There was no garden, but I knew we could make money by renting out some of the rooms. I said to Pauline that we could have two floors for ourselves to live in and we could rent out the other four floors and make enough money to pay the mortgage and make some savings. Then perhaps ten years later we could buy another house and still have an income from the Chelsham Road house.

I did not get the usually supportive response I was expecting. Pauline looked at me and said: 'So you expect me to spend the best ten years of my life, with two babies to bring up, living with tenants!' She was clearly horrified by my clever plan. 'How are you going to give me back those ten years of happiness?' she asked me. I realised that I was completely wrong with my money-making plan: she needed her garden and her home and I learned there and then, if I did not already know it perfectly well, how much wiser than myself was my wife. Of course I could never give her back those ten years of happiness. Other things can be more valuable than money and it is important never to be completely ruled by it. Pauline and I were firm friends long before we became romantically involved and I think that has been very important for us: friendship is so important because if you are good friends you will always like each other.

Pauline remembers rejecting the chance to return to Chelsham Road:

I completely freaked when Toni came up with the idea. I said, 'You must be joking!' – I didn't want other people living in our family house. But to be fair to Toni, he had been used to living like that with lots of lodgers and people renting rooms. He tried for a few days to convince me but I was not having it and he agreed. However, with another baby on the way we did need more space. I went round the estate agents and found a lovely big semi-detached house for sale in nearby Streatham. It was perfect – we had a new house and our lovely little daughter and soon we were to have another new baby, our beautiful son Christian. Unlike Sacha he never cried and was always so calm and laid-back.

We had been very happy in 146 King's Avenue, Clapham but it really was only a little cottage. We used to say that it was like a doll's house. We sold it for about £12,000 and the house that Pauline found, 25 Abbotswood Road, Streatham, cost £21,000. It was much bigger, probably double the size of our first home together. The rooms were huge and it had five bedrooms. Later we put an extension on the back and knocked two rooms into one downstairs to make a lovely big living room. It was very spacious, and a beautiful place after we had done it up.

My memories of the early years of our marriage are of enormous happiness mixed with great tiredness. I was so pleased and proud to be a husband to Pauline and a father to little Sacha, even if she did cry a lot, and to our second little miracle, Christian. Family has always been so important to me all my life and now I was the head of one of my own; it felt so right. But there was always a lot of work to do. The salons were very busy, fortunately, and I was still doing all the paperwork as well as working all day cutting and styling hair, six long days a week. I tried to help Pauline when I got home and so often we were both exhausted but there was still some time for a little social life, even if it sometimes came at inconvenient moments.

One of those times came in 1972, on 6 May. It was my thirtieth birthday, and I was feeling pretty bad and certainly not at all like celebrating. I was suffering with a horrible toothache, but I was still smiling away at the clients as I worked away in Clapham. I was again suffering very badly with my gums and all the treatment I had was penicillin and then more penicillin. Then out of the blue my friend Michael Stylianou came in. He said he just happened to be passing and had just called in to say 'Hello'. *That's nice of him,* I thought and when he suggested we went to the pub for a drink

I could hardly refuse. It was the last thing I felt like because I had a headache as well as the toothache. I was really suffering and I thought, *God, he would have to come today!* I liked to see him, but I really didn't feel well.

I said I wasn't well and just wanted to go home to bed. He said: 'No, no, no! I'll give you a lift home.' Normally Pauline used to come and pick me up as we only had one car at the time. Of course we had to have a quick beer on the way and then when we arrived home there was a big surprise party for my birthday. It was a very happy occasion in the end and I even started to forget about my headache and my toothache. It was also the first of many surprise parties. I am fortunate to have had a lot of them all the way through my life. I thought it was really nice to see lots of family and friends, some of whom I hadn't seen for a long time. It was certainly a sign for the future. Pauline has always been amazing at springing surprise parties on me, probably because she knows perfectly well that if I was asked beforehand whether or not I wanted a party, I'd definitely say no!

We had a much more serious problem later in 1972 with the birth of Christian. For Sacha's birth the doctor at Dulwich Hospital was very, very good, but he was on holiday when Christian arrived in August. Christian was a very big baby and there was no doctor on duty at the hospital, just a midwife. It was terrible for Pauline because they needed someone to do a Caesarean and there was no one around. Poor Pauline was in awful agony and after the ordeal she became anaemic. For a long, long time she had no energy whatsoever. For example, on Christmas Eve she would try to prepare everything for the perfect family Christmas and then it would be all too much for her and she would just faint. Her willpower was very, very strong but the energy was just not there.

Many times I used to have to pick her up off the floor and put her to bed.

Pauline can never forget the trauma of the birth of her second baby:

Christian's birth turned into a terrifying emergency. I nearly died having him. I was eight months pregnant when I was rushed into hospital. I was put on a heart machine at one point. They should have done a Caesarean but they didn't, so I was still in a bit of a state after I came out of hospital with the baby. I had Sacha, who was just a year and a couple of months old, and this tiny baby to care for. God must have been looking over me because Sacha stopped crying as soon as her little brother arrived home and Christian was a very good and easy baby.

Sacha was remarkable. Even when she was very young she wanted to be like a little mum for Christian. She loved him so much I am sure that is why she stopped crying. But I was very ill and so weak I could hardly do anything for a long time. I was backwards and forwards to the hospital having tests done and then I had to have an operation. Times were hard and it was especially hard for Toni. My parents stepped in and so did my sister – they were always there for me. My dad had lost a sister who died in childbirth and he hated me having children because he was so scared he might lose me. But my sister took it all in her stride. It was a piece of cake to her, in spite of looking after her own big family. I was ill for six or seven years after having Christian and I was always very concerned about the children. I made sure they were with me at all times possible. I never wanted to let them out of my sight – I always felt frightened that something would happen to them. The memory of Toni losing his mum was always there.

After the operation I got a bit better but for ten years I wasn't well. Then, before I fell pregnant with Pierre, I had to go and have all these tests done and they found I had a germ in my blood – a virus associated with glandular fever – and they couldn't get rid of it, and it is still there, today. Some days I wake up and I just can't do anything, which I hate because I am normally a very busy person, but you learn to relax and go into yourself.

I suppose Pauline is right: I did worry a lot, and if I am totally honest it was a deep sense of insecurity that drove me on to work so hard. I was determined never to let my family down and the only way I knew was to work very, very hard so I could look after them.

Strong family values have influenced my whole life very deeply and they are still all-important to me today. I am very lucky that two wonderful women have helped to instil those values, my mother and the woman who became my wife. Of course they are completely different people from completely different countries but they share many great qualities, from kindness and loyalty to total honesty and the ability to create the happiest of homes.

I was a very lucky man a long time before I became successful.

CHAPTER SIX

INTO THE
WEST END: MAYFAIR

The early seventies were a time of great change and sustained turbulence for my family and me, for my adopted country and indeed for the wider world. War raged in Vietnam, terrorists struck at the Munich Olympics, the IRA brought terrible conflict to the streets of Britain and a chilling economic disaster loomed just as our fledgling family business really began to find its feet. The crippling paralysis of the three-day week was hardly the time to launch a brave new enterprise but often in business it is the moment that seizes you rather than the other way round.

Yet as the decade began prospects looked bright for the future. We had three shops that were all busy and we were getting increasingly better off financially, although we worked very hard. We built up a very healthy number of regular customers, many of whom became friends for life. Lots of actresses lived in the areas near our salons and we had famous faces from *Coronation Street* and many other TV shows and films in our chairs. They seemed to like the bustling family atmosphere that was always a natural but hugely important part of our service.

When I was first married, with a daughter and a son arriving very quickly was a time when I found my friendly financial adviser, Mr Feak, to be a particularly great support. Mr Feak was an exceptional person. Possibly because he had spent time in Italy during the war he had absolutely fallen in love with the country of my birth and its people. He spoke perfect Italian with a strong English accent, and was a typical officer of the British Army in his mannerisms. Very honest and supportive, he was always ready to help you in every way. He looked after me and almost all of the Italian restaurateurs and other businessmen in London. Lots of them couldn't speak English very well and he insured their houses, cars and organised their private pensions. He was a friend to everybody, loved by all and to me he was more than a friend, he was almost like a second father.

Often he would come to my house in the evening to talk about different ways he could help me with the family. He was most kind and always complimentary about everything. A great motivator, he set a good example for me to follow. With his help I began to learn a little about making money with money. With just a few bits of savings I realised it was going to be impossible to be able to afford to pay for my children's private education so I invested in a ten-year endowment policy that was tax deductible with profits. As it matured I would be able to afford the school fees, I took one out every two years, with each one to mature at two-year intervals. The costs were minimal and I was able to get best education for my children.

My friend Michael Stylianou offered me an even more direct way of saving money when he took me to a cash-and-carry warehouse for the first time. In those days, before large supermarkets dominated the retail scene, the prices demanded by local corner shops for basic necessities such as milk or sugar were relatively high. Food was very expensive then. Michael showed me there were large savings to be made by buying from the cash-and-carry outlets, especially if you bought in bulk.

I have always loved saving money and I quickly found that if I arrived by car, or better still, in a borrowed van I could buy everything from nappies and disinfectant to salt and canned food at very good prices. Often it was a 100 per cent cheaper. It was just amazing. *OK, I'll start building up my supplies,* I thought. Not only would it save me money, it saved me time because I didn't have to do my shopping every single week. Instead I went six times a year, which saved me a lot of hassle. I would buy enough salt, sugar and other non-perishables to last me a year. I bought all the household things that would keep a long time. You could also buy good-quality meat as the outlet owners had their own farms. I would buy a whole lamb and they would cut it up for me to put in the freezer – it was a very good way to save money. I used to go five or six times a year and I could save enough money to take the whole family on holiday to Italy. My motto in life has always been: If you respect money, you will always have money. The same goes for your friends: If you respect your friends, you will always have friends.

All my life I have been very careful with money. I have always conserved money and tried to make it work for me when I can. At this time I knew nothing about buying shares on the stock market but I kept reading of certain dramatic rises and people making large profits, thanks to choosing the right company to invest in. I turned to the dependable Mr Feak to see if he could advise me on which shares to choose.

In his sternest voice he said to me: 'How much money have you saved, Toni?' I said I had about £100 available and he replied: 'Good. Go and hire yourself a van, which will cost you about £5. Then take all the cash you have and go to the wholesaler and spend it all there.' Clearly Michael Stylianou was right. Mr Feak said: 'You will get the equivalent of 300 per cent earnings, guaranteed at the wholesaler. Forget the stock market, put it completely out of your head because you could lose all your money in a moment.' It was very good advice and I have never forgotten it.

Anthony left school in 1972 and went to work in the Streatham salon with my father. He was very artistic and very talented and a great addition to the family team. For a while he lived with us in Abbotswood Road. Pauline recalls:

I loved having Anthony with us, but it was hard for him and not always easy for us. In some ways he had thought of me as his mum and now I had young children of my own. Anthony was a teenager, it was difficult – there were a few times when I had to scour the streets for him when he was out late!

It was now almost ten years since we had first begun trading as Toni & Guy in Clapham and much had changed in that time. A decade of hard work had established our family business, but I knew that to really succeed and to establish ourselves as leading London hairdressers we needed to move to the centre of the city. We had lots of ambition and great belief in our abilities, but we were never going to fulfil our potential with three salons in Clapham, Streatham and Mitcham.

We had the talent, of that I had no doubt. But as my brothers and I began to use photographs to promote our work it was clear that no one really wanted to publicise a suburban salon. It is also the case that the area around the salons was changing with a huge influx of immigrants moving into that part of south London, including many from the Caribbean. With my Italian background and English home and family I do not believe I am guilty of racism, but the number of new arrivals was too great to be easily assimilated. It was like introducing a nation into a nation when they arrived all at the same time.

We knew things were bad but we didn't realise what a huge economic crisis was about to grip us and the whole country when the Government started printing petrol-rationing books in November 1973, and just before Christmas our Prime Minister, Mr Edward Heath, unveiled the grim news of the 'three-day week'. As union disputes paralysed industry and oil costs spiralled, it was announced that businesses would be allowed to have electricity for only three days of their normal working week. With our six-day operation this meant half our hairdressing had to be conducted in what natural light there was in the gloomiest months of the year. It became known as the Winter of Discontent and it was certainly a very difficult time for us. Our salons were always bright and full of light and energy. It was not easy at times but we just carried on, working as hard as we could and endeavouring to please our clients. There were lots of power cuts and many times the whirr of the hairdryers would suddenly stop and the lights would go out.

Fortunately for us, my father's salons back in Scafati had often suffered from an intermittent power supply so that experience meant that we were more able to adapt than many others. He had passed on various styling and drying techniques that would overcome the sudden lack of power. And it was often very atmospheric in a candlelit salon. Whatever happened to the electricity supply, we were determined that the work would go ahead. We had no choice, really.

London was changing enormously at this time. Millions of people from all over the globe came to visit the city, which was clearly becoming the capital of the world. Americans and Japanese flocked here, followed by people from every country on the planet. Everyone wanted to see Carnaby Street and the rest of the sights as the cultural reverberations from the Swinging Sixties resounded on well into the astonishing seventies. People wanted to see the latest fashions for themselves. The desire too for education in every detail of the newest trends was international. Bruno and Anthony were bursting to display their talents on the biggest stages possible and Guy and I accepted that while we had built the foundations of a business in south London, the time had come to move to the centre.

Of course my brothers wanted to arrive in the West End instantly, but it was not so easy as that. I searched hard for the right place, revisiting my old haunts in Mayfair and Knightsbridge and marvelling at how much London's most fashionable districts had altered in just a few short years. The old village atmosphere had long gone and with an ever-growing premium on price there was a real shortage of suitable sites for a stylish Italian hairdresser to set up shop. I spent a lot of time driving round in the evening, searching for somewhere for us to establish ourselves. From our first ten years I had saved as much money as I could for this great leap forward but I had long since learned that the right property always comes at a high price.

First I tried for a place in Knightsbridge, just off Sloane Street. It was a promising location on the first floor with its own entrance, but we lost it by a whisker. It was frustrating but it just didn't happen and I had to start again. Then another place came up. I found Number 12, Davies Street, where an old Jewish man called Harold had run a hairdressing salon for years – it seemed then that every hairdresser in the United Kingdom was Jewish. We must have been the first Catholic ones. Harold didn't mind at all, he was quite flashy and outspoken. He had been successful and built up a good clientele, mostly from the immediate area, and now he wanted to retire.

We talked and he seemed to warm to the idea of selling the business to us, but the landlords, as with so many of the properties in that area, were the Grosvenor Estate. Old and traditional, they were very English in their attitude and did not seem all that excited by the prospect of giving a lease to young Italian boys with no connections. Fortunately, Harold wanted to do a deal with us and he was extremely helpful. He was a very feminine kind of guy and with hindsight I suppose he was gay, although in those days I'm not sure we recognised that. He liked me and my brothers and he worked hard to persuade the landlords to give us a chance. We signed the lease and it cost much, much more than the £20 a week we had started off with in Clapham. It was more like £20,000 a year but it turned out to be a very good deal.

We sold the Mitcham and Streatham salons to help finance the move to Davies Street, even though I was totally against that decision. I always remember my father telling me never to sell and always to buy and that was in the back of my mind. He and I were of the same opinion even then. I didn't want to sell anything – I thought they were assets that would appreciate anyway over time but Bruno insisted and so I relented and let him have his way. We sold the Mitcham business first and then a few months later we also sold the salon in Streatham.

We were in Mayfair, in the heart of the West End, only a hundred yards from Berkeley Square. To me it was frightening because of the cost, but at the same time very exciting. We decorated the outside of our new establishment in brown and cream and opened our doors in autumn 1974. The design was very funky and at that time many of the styles of the twenties were experiencing a revival so we launched the salon before receiving a chastening surprise. It was very, very quiet at first. One or two of our faithful customers from Clapham, Streatham or Mitcham did make the journey to see our new establishment but at first clients were extremely thin on the ground. Fortunately the photographs of our work came to the rescue. The free news magazines, *Ms London* and *Girl About Town*, were handed out on street corners all over the capital. We advertised some of our styles and with our all-important W1 address, it proved very effective. Within a few weeks we were mercifully busy and it seemed our great gamble might have a chance of paying off. We were quite close to the Italian Embassy and very soon the Ambassador and a lot of his staff were coming in regularly.

I held the fort in Clapham, which was still a very profitable business with a strong clientele that had been built over ten years, while my brothers and my father built up the business in Davies Street. Unfortunately I could only go to Davies Street for a small part of every week because most of the time I was working hard in Clapham. The £20-a-week rent had become cheap, thanks to inflation. We were very, very busy and made more money there than ever before. Thank God for that because things had started to go from bad to worse in the economy and I was very pleased to have kept that very good income so that I could support the growth of the Davies Street, which was salon still not breaking even. But after a short time it started to grow rapidly and began to be profitable.

The potential was incredible and it needed my full involvement; my brothers encouraged me to leave Clapham and to be in Davies Street full time. I continued to look after all of the accounts and purchases for Clapham and for Davies Street. It was an incredibly busy time for me and I continued to use all of my free time to work and to keep a full column of clients and help as much as possible. I convinced Pauline to help and run the business as she had an amazing relationship with all of the staff and they adored her. There was a mutual respect and it was a great opportunity and extremely rewarding for Pauline; she could have easily bought her dream car, a Mercedes, in a very short time with the profits. She hardly had any expenses and the salon business was very profitable. It worked a dream.

Sacha and Christian were now at nursery school and she still spent a lot of time with them but deep down she wanted to just look after her children. That was her first love and everything came to a head when Sacha said to her: 'Oh, Mummy, why can't you be like all the other mummies and be at home all the time with me?' Not that she was neglecting her at all. Sacha was always well cared for, but it had a profound impact on my wife. I first heard about it when Pauline came in one morning and out of the blue said: 'You are disgusting – you only think about making money but my family comes first!'

I just thought, *My God, all this money lost.* So I had to put a manager in for Clapham. I found an extremely personable guy called John, who seemed very competent and was popular with the ladies. I thought he would do well and for a while he did. He kept the salon going and when I was there he worked very hard and the salon was always full. When I was busy in Davies Street I used to phone him regularly to keep a check on him and he always said he was busy. Yet I soon noticed that the salon turnover was dropping alarmingly. So I decided to investigate and I went to Clapham and worked there for a couple of days. I met clients who told me they were sorry that they had not been able to get booked in. To my horror John was turning many of our faithful customers away. He had a very different philosophy to mine: he was so lazy, he only did 20 per cent of the clients! I could not believe he was actually turning people away. I never like losing staff but this time there was no alternative so I fired him. I felt angry and badly let down but it soon transpired that he was only a minor setback compared with the economic crisis that was about to grip us and the whole country.

One of our great strengths was our originality. We never copied anyone else, we always preferred to design and develop our own styles. In Davies Street we started with a chunky look, which was the complete opposite of what Vidal Sassoon was doing with all his geometric cuts. Although my brothers and I disagreed on many, many things in our decades together, we always agreed that we wanted to go our own way. We never wanted to follow what someone else was doing; we always wanted to create our own styles. We loved using very feminine, very Italian hairstyles for our clients. It was an extremely exciting time and the great thing was that many of our clients shared our enthusiasm. Those chunky cuts with lots of curls eventually found their way to the actresses who starred in *Charlie's Angels*. We also created the famous Purdey style featured on Joanna Lumley in *The New Avengers*.

Unfortunately we didn't really get the credit for creating these hugely popular styles that went on to be so popular on television because everyone was able to copy our designs as soon as they saw them. In this country at that time if you wanted to do a special style for television you had to have a union card. We didn't have one and we had no way of getting one. The Americans used to come over and learn all our haircuts and then recreate them for actresses back in America. So we would look at *Dallas* when it arrived on television and see all the twisted plaits and other distinctive styles first seen at Toni & Guy. Everyone thought these amazing new designs came from America but in fact many of them came from Toni & Guy. It became the heart of hairdressing. The popularity of the salon grew and grew. It was an amazing time and often we were overwhelmed by the response.

We were very fortunate with our next move, because just as we were bursting at the seams with clients, the premises next door, which had housed an art gallery, became available. It was handy being next door so we decided to buy the lease, which we managed very quickly, and soon we had another immaculate salon. It was extremely convenient even if you did have to go out of the front door on to the pavement to get from one salon to the other! My father insisted this was crazy. He could not see why on earth we should have to go outside to move from one part of the business to another. I tried to explain that the building belonged to the Grosvenor Estate, who would almost certainly veto any drastic structural changes, but he was not in the mood for listening. Instead he said: 'That's totally stupid. Leave it to me.'

That evening, after everyone had gone home, he went in with a big hammer and knocked a huge hole in the wall between the two properties. Then he got one of his friends to install an RSJ (a steel joist to support the wall) to make it safe, and when we all arrived at work the next morning there was a great big doorway between the two shops. My father just stood there next to it, smiled and said: 'You see, now it's much simpler. You can go straight through!'

I was horrified. 'Oh my God! What have you done? Now they're going to kick us out,' I said. I was sure this would mean big trouble from our landlords because I knew the Grosvenor Estate were very strict in the way they administered their property and I was pretty sure that you were not allowed to knock a great big hole in a wall whenever you felt like it. All these years later it is still the same today so my father's direct action paid off. We did ask for retrospective permission from Grosvenor and in the end we agreed that we would reinstate the wall and remove my dad's doorway whenever we left. Happily that hasn't happened yet and the doorway helped us a great deal. It brought the two salons much more together and we ended up with a 60-seater salon that kept thirty-two hairdressers busy. It was a big place but soon it would prove not big enough as business boomed.

My father had great confidence in everything he did. I think he was the most optimistic person I've ever known. One one occasion, we – my father, Guy and myself – were going to see a lawyer in Lincoln's Inn. We were supposed to be there at 12 o'clock, but we did not get into our car, parked on Chesham Road in Clapham, until about 11.45. We turned into Wandsworth Road to find it totally blocked. In those days there was a huge campaign against Mr Marples: 'Marples must go!' said the posters. He was the Minister of Transport and it must have been a popular campaign since all the roads seemed totally jammed. This was long before the one-way system. It was obvious we were going to be late. I complained that this would cost us more money (always I was the one who worried about the practical things in life). We were going to talk about a piece of land in Italy. My father was quite a wheeler-dealer at times. He said: 'We'll get there on time, I promise you. Why are you always so worried?' Anyway, the lawyer's time was not important to my father. He wasn't at all concerned about being late because he knew he could win him over with his excuses. Of course we were now very late but my father couldn't care less; even after 12 o'clock he insisted we would be on time. In spite of our horrendous lateness, we did get to see the lawyer, who I remember wore very thick silver-framed glasses. My dad was quite a character, and I believe some of his powerful positive thinking eventually rubbed off on me.

I was blessed with having much hugely artistic talent in my family and Bruno and Anthony were particularly keen on doing shows to demonstrate our hairdressing skills in the most entertaining way possible. We worked with a brilliant chap called Renato Brunas, who helped stage these shows at a time when he was launching his own company. He had excellent entrepreneurial skills and it was great to work with him. I remember when Renato launched Crazy Color – he came up with very strong, extreme colours that were quite unique in the market at that time.

Renato used to bring furniture over from Italy and he was one of the first hairdressing entrepreneurs of the time. He was trying to challenge the big established colour companies; he was very together and he helped lift us to the next level. We started creating all these new, strong and powerful looks, from typically feminine, commercial chunky layers to a mixture of geometric cuts. It was the time when we combined the British geometric and precise cutting with the soft, feminine Italian look – that really seemed to grab a lot of interest from the public. We did a special curly perm as well, which we called 'wash and leave'. All these types of hairstyle were very commercial and easy to manage. We were all very much on the same wavelength: we believed in what we were doing and that we had new styles that would be really popular. And of course I always felt Guy was the most artistic salon hairdresser that ever lived. Very popular with all of the clients, he was always a charmer, always available, and would try anything that his client wanted. Extremely artistic and unique in the world of hairdressing, he had a waiting list of clients who were prepared to wait several weeks for an appointment, but at the same time he was a very quick salon hairdresser and would do thirty to thirty-five clients a day, some waiting hours on end for his touch.

The photographs in the magazines and in leaflets we put out certainly had clients coming in droves to our salons. The only trouble was they boosted lots of rival hairdressers as well. One of the directors of Robert Fielding, who had about twenty-five salons in London, passed by our salon one day and came in to thank me. He brought in an armful of our photos and leaflets featuring our style and said to me: 'You have made me a fortune, sir. I have made so much money, I have sold the company!' He then moved to California. Not surprisingly he was very happy indeed.

Everybody wanted our fantastic hairstyles and we had only the two shops. We worked as hard as we could, but lots of people went to other hairdressers with pictures of our styles cut from the magazines. That really started me thinking. I thought, *Wow, he has done really well out of me,* but that was how it was. I knew we needed to do something else to develop our full potential.

We decided we should show people our ideas and our styles so we set out on putting together our first book of hairdressing styles. I wanted to show the world what we had created and I soon realised that selling the books was another way to make money.

People wanted to know how to do our hairstyles and I decided we should also make videotapes of the cutting and styling to show exactly how we did things. We made both VHS and Betamax videos featuring about forty different types of style for different lengths of hair. Unfortunately we were ahead of our time because there were not enough tape machines on the market as the demand was so high. Consumers couldn't purchase video players as they had completely sold out!

Our reputation grew very quickly and lots of people took an interest in Toni & Guy. Vidal Sassoon had been the most famous name in hairdressing but soon we at Toni & Guy were up there at the forefront alongside him. We had many very famous people in our salon. The composer Andrew Lloyd Webber used to come in a lot and so did the Australian comedian Barry Humphries, singers Diana Ross and Dana, Hollywood actor Gregory Peck, and countless others; Guy used to do the Duke of Westminster's secretary's hair as well. But they all got exactly the same treatment as a lady who walked in off the street because our philosophy was, and still is today, that all clients are special, and we treated everyone exactly the same.

A very gifted young hairdresser called Trevor Sorbie was made artistic director for Vidal Sassoon in 1973 and after a while he was keen to come and work with us. Sassoon was very well established and popular, but we were the new kids on the block and Sorbie was particularly keen to work with my younger brothers. Already he had quite a name but he knew he needed more experience. A fantastic hairdresser, he was very strong and confident, and he did the wedge, which soon became very famous. He was a highly talented young man and Pauline was delighted with the way he did her hair a few times. But he was more of an artist than a strong commercial salon hairdresser and after about eighteen months he moved on to develop his career, as we knew he would.

We were four brothers on an exciting journey with our business. Each of us had talent and lots of ideas and lots of energy. We wanted to do lots of things. Every night we would have a meeting after work and I would be like the officer in charge, a field marshal if you like, directing operations and trying to make sure everyone did the right thing. We talked about our hopes and ambitions all the time; we were young and impatient to go places. But I was the one who had to convert all this wild enthusiasm and different personalities into a business.

My brother Guy was always much more relaxed than me. He once went to sleep in a board meeting! Another time he came to me to tell me about a lady client who had a restaurant in Victoria called La Signora di Victoria. She was a large and successful lady and her husband was a real gentleman, said Guy. But what had most impressed him was that she used to work for just six months of the year in the restaurant and then spend the other six months on holiday in Italy, while her brother ran the restaurant. After six months it would be her brother's turn for half a year's holiday.

Guy said: 'This is brilliant! This is what we can achieve – we can each have six months' holiday every year.' I was excited myself for a while about that. At first I thought it was indeed brilliant but then I started to think more deeply about the idea. I realised that after six months' holiday we would not present a challenge to other hairdressers. It is an extremely fast-moving business and I realised we would lose our competitive edge. We would lose touch with our customers, who all had their favourite hairdresser. We would not be flying any longer; instead we would just have been plodding along. I think we were too young for that. And also, to be honest, I didn't really want to have six months off because I love my work. I still do, and I still don't want six months off, even today.

Guy was always one to work very, very hard in bursts and then take it easy. My trademark has always been consistency. I believed then and I believe now in building slowly and steadily. We still had a terrific amount of excitement together; the salon was a hive of activity. My financial friend Jack Feak put it best when he arrived one day in our salon in Davies Street on a Saturday afternoon, which was our busiest time, and there was not a seat empty in the whole salon. There were people everywhere and he boomed out: 'Toni, Toni, I've come through Grosvenor Square, Berkeley Square and all through Mayfair and there was not a soul about! I couldn't understand it until I came into your salon – they're all in here!'

What a great compliment from one of my great helpers.

★　★　★

My brother Bruno was always full of ideas. Some of them were great and others were not so great, but right from the time he joined us he was keenly focused on the visual potential of our business. He thought of hairdressers not just as simple stylists but also performers, even in the early days. Back in 1969, shortly after we had opened our third salon, he had come up with the brainwave of staging a live fashion show with a strong hairdressing theme. At the time Bruno said: 'If we perform close to our new salon in Mitcham not only will it be good local publicity, but it may also spread our name a little further afield.'

The show went on in a nearby church hall and Bruno and Guy were up on stage flamboyantly doing their stuff while the music of Marvin Gaye blasted round the building. The audience was mainly made up of teenage girls who went crazy over the styles and also took a keen interest in my brothers. It was a successful event and it helped to show us all that there was real hope for the future in the family business.

Bruno was always the easiest of my brothers to clash with and we had many, many disagreements. Most of them were not personal and easily resolved, but it was not so quickly forgotten when we fell out over his wedding in 1974. I didn't go because I had already booked a family holiday to Cyprus with my friend Michael and his family. Bruno thought I should have changed my holiday but I didn't want to do that, particularly after the hardships of the 'three-day week'. It was unfortunate because little Sacha was to be his bridesmaid but he refused to change the date of the wedding. In the end the holiday was changed to Corfu because war broke out on Cyprus between the Greeks and the Turks, but I was very disappointed for my daughter and not being at his wedding upset me tremendously.

By the time we were established in Davies Street we were in a period of great change. Many older styles of business were being hastily revamped and reorganised. I knew that, with our Italian family culture, our hairdressing abilities and our growing reputation we had to come up with new ways of building and developing Toni & Guy. In my mind the one word I kept coming back to was education, education, education. It seemed like a natural progression, when you have created this level of interest and reputation with magazine photographs and quality hairdressing, for us to show our clients and the public at large more of our talents. More and more people were asking how we created styles and what was going to be the next popular craze to sweep the nation so I started the idea of us delivering seminars to show the world how to do it.

I turned initially to a very talented young man called Anestis Cobella. He was a Greek Cypriot boy who had worked with me in Clapham with his sister, after my brothers had moved to Davies Street. They were nice, hard-working people who really wanted to get on in life. Anestis's sister was a very good hairdresser and she stayed with me in Clapham while he later moved on to work with my brothers. He was very involved with putting on shows and then we started doing seminars, downstairs at Davies Street, on Sundays and Mondays.

Bruno started the seminars and after a while Anestis became our seminar director. We were very busy putting on shows, doing videos, preparing books and seminars, as well as handling the day-to-day business of running extremely busy salons. Bruno was quick to see the potential in running seminars; he was always very clever and always motivated and encouraged others to get involved and to become teachers. The only trouble is that when you get other people to do things for you they sometimes get to the point where they want to move on and do things for themselves. Anestis met a stunning English girl, Beverly, and then said he needed to marry her to be able to stay in Britain. I remember him saying to her: 'Look, I will marry you because I want to stay in this country!' I was shocked and I said to Anestis: 'Are you crazy? She is beautiful! You should marry her, certainly, but not just because you want to stay in the country. Tell her you want to marry her because you love her!'

After they married, she and Anestis started their own company, Cobella Hairdressing, which became very successful. Beverly was very, very good at the job and was British Hairdresser of the Year a couple of times. Later, when she and her husband came to a parting of the ways, she worked with me for a while, before going on to set up her own business. Anestis and I remain friends to this day and I still see him often.

★ ★ ★

Later we decided we should create a proper hairdressing school within Toni & Guy. I searched for a suitable location for a school but in the meantime decided to take advantage of the basement space we had in Davies Street. We found a space for six students to come in for a complete week's training in advanced styling. It cost £1,200, so it made money for the company from the very start. We had a small television and we used our own videos as part of the course. We employed a teacher who had come from an established school and was already experienced in teaching as well as being a talented artist. I paid him £200 a week, which was very good pay in those days. By using our existing facilities and products there was no real extra cost to the business. It was a big success – the courses were booked up for weeks and then even months ahead. Demand was really building but then the teacher had a car accident and lost all of his confidence, which was a setback. But while it was running the course made £1,000 a week. That is £50,000 a year clear profit, which was great for the business. It was fantastic! We ran it for about a year before I realised we needed somewhere bigger and so I started looking for separate premises for our first academy.

With a young family and a demanding business there never seemed to be enough hours in the day to achieve all my aims. Fortunately I was blessed with plenty of energy and I was always very driven but even so there are events in life that really knock you out of your stride. My father's sudden early death on 18

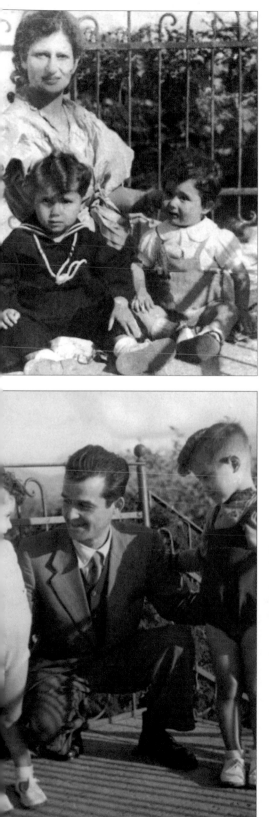

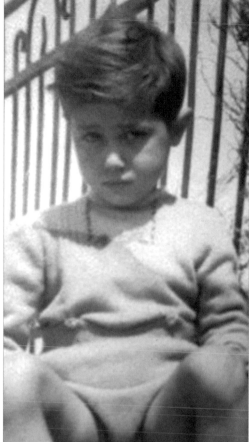

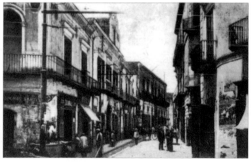

Above left: My mother, Maria, with me and Guy, probably in about 1946.

© *Toni Mascolo*

Above right: Me, aged six, in Italy, looking very angry during a session with a professional photographer. © *Toni Mascolo*

Below left: With my father and Guy *(left)* in 1948. © *Toni Mascolo*

Below right: Humble beginnings – a shot of the street where I grew up in Scafati.

© *Toni Mascolo*

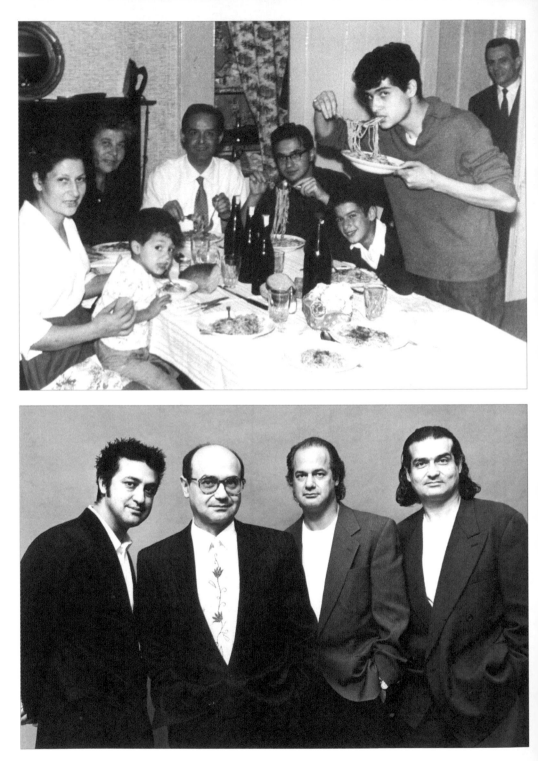

Above: A typical Italian family supper at 59 Chelsham Road – from left to right, my mother with Anthony, an aunt who was visiting from Italy, my father, myself, Bruno and Guy.

©*Toni Mascolo*

Below: 'The Beatles of Hairdressing' – from left to right, Anthony, me, Bruno and Guy in the 1990s.

© *Toni Mascolo*

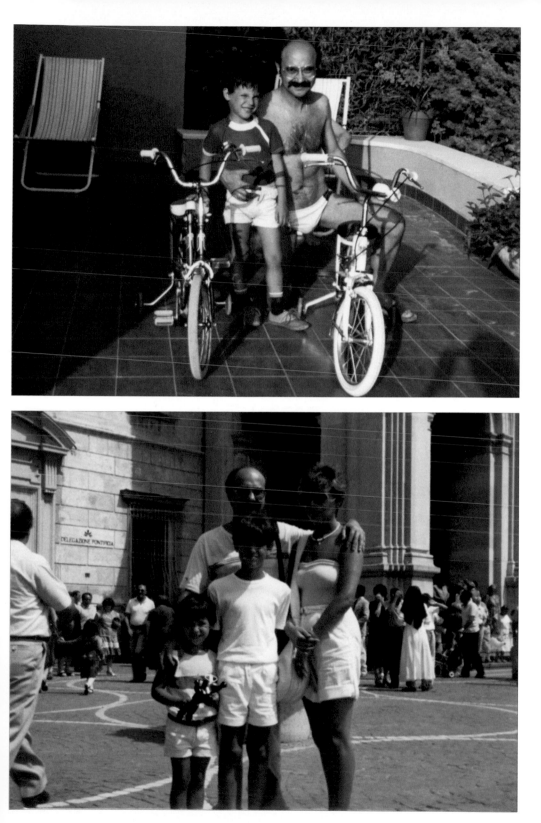

Enjoying a family holiday in Pompeii, 1985, with Pauline and my sons, Christian and Pierre.

© Toni Mascolo

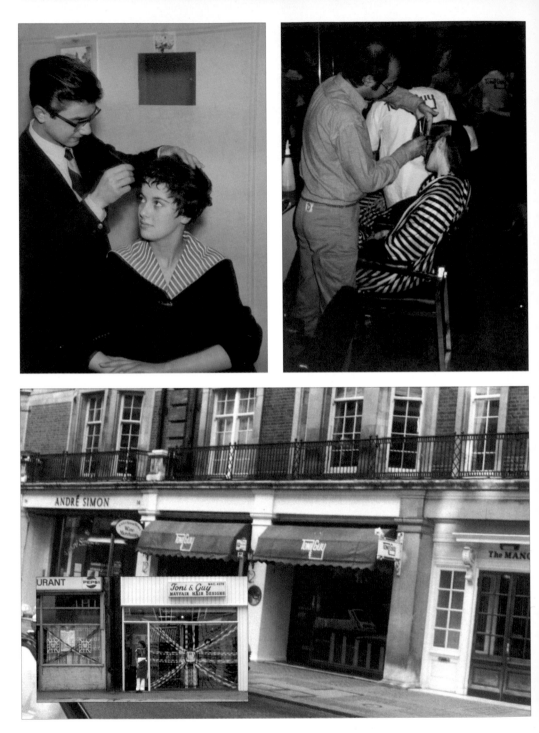

Above left: I began cutting people's hair at the tender age of fifteen. © *Toni Mascolo*

Above right: Me at a hairdressing show in Wembley in 1977. © *Toni Mascolo*

Inset: 40 Clapham Park Road – the very first Toni & Guy salon. It was here that I met my beloved wife, Pauline. © *Toni Mascolo*

Below: 12 Davies Street in 1974 – our first Mayfair salon and an exciting new direction for Toni & Guy. © *Toni Mascolo*

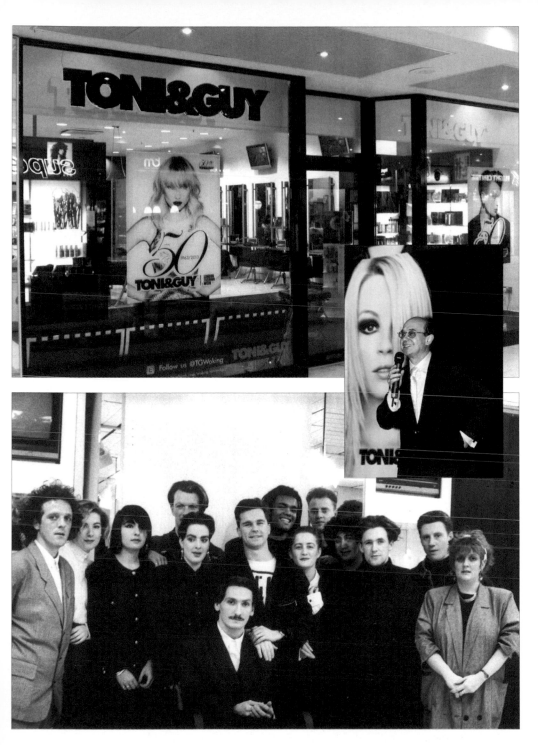

Above: From a small shop in Clapham to a global franchise – a Toni & Guy salon today.

© *Toni Mascolo*

Inset: I was proud to celebrate four decades of Toni & Guy in 2003.

© *Toni Mascolo*

Below: The Toni & Guy family – we have been running academies and seminars since the early 1970s and this is a team from the early 80s. Today we have more than 8,000 employees across the world.

© *Toni Mascolo*

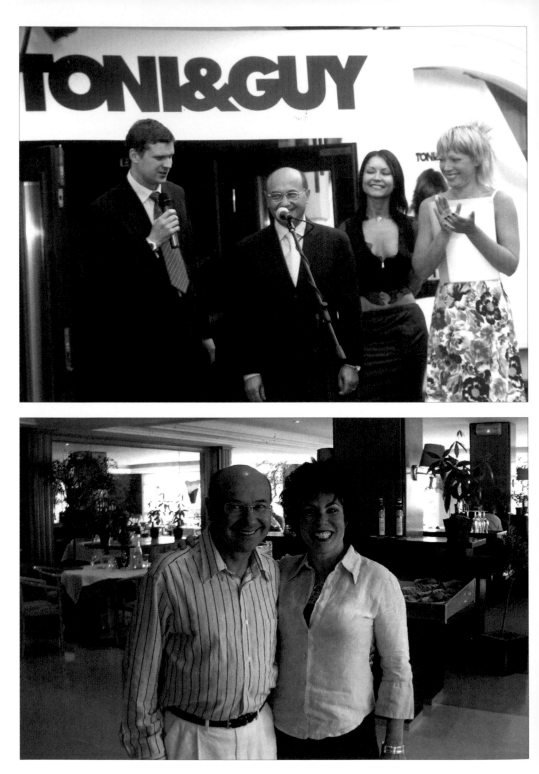

Above: Going global – visiting Moscow in 2002. © *Toni Mascolo*

Below: Ruby Wax tried hard to dish the dirt on us when she made a television programme about Toni & Guy in 2004, but there was simply none to be found.

© *Toni Mascolo*

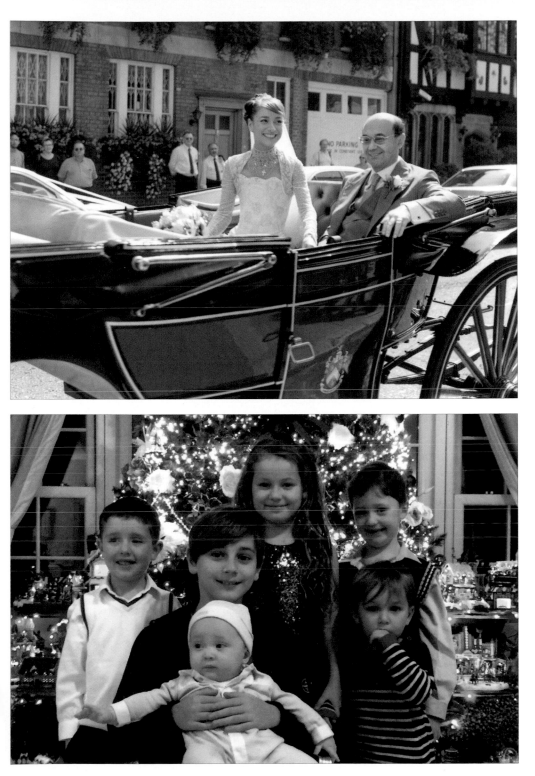

Above: Family will always come first for me. Here I am with my beautiful daughter, Sacha (a talented hairdresser and businesswoman in her own right), on her wedding day in August 2001.

© *Toni Mascolo*

Below: I am also a proud grandfather of six.

© *Toni Mascolo*

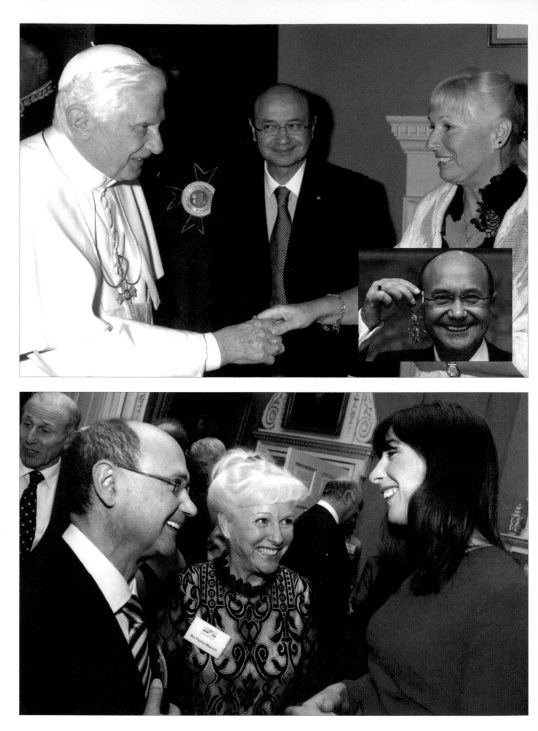

Above: Pauline and I were deeply moved to be presented with a Papal Knighthood in March 2013. © *Toni Mascolo*

Inset: Although I was a little disappointed not to have been awarded this by the Queen, I was still absolutely thrilled to be appointed an honorary OBE in 2008. © *Toni Mascolo*

Below: Pauline and I have been lucky enough to meet many marvellous people over the years, including Samantha Cameron in 2010. © *Toni Mascolo*

December 1976 was one of the most shocking of those events. We learned later that he was desperately ill with cancer, but he had carefully kept the severity of his condition from all of us brothers so the news came as a complete bombshell.

He was only sixty-two years old, much too young to die, and we were all absolutely devastated. Back in 1965, on a typically busy evening in Clapham, with the salon full of clients, my father came down the stairs and slightly twisted his ankle. We asked if he was OK and if he wanted to sit down. We were all joking and teasing him and we asked if he wanted us to call an ambulance. To our shock and surprise he said yes and that was when we realised he was really hurt. So we called an ambulance. He seemed to recover from that but then he became ill and ended up in hospital, where he was diagnosed with cancer.

I was desperately upset and so too were all my brothers and everyone in the family. I felt it was a delayed reaction to the death of my mother. He was then taken to a hospice, where terminal patients go to end their days. The doctor told us it was a hospice, but we didn't tell my father. Perhaps not surprisingly, he was horrified by the mortality rate of his fellow patients. When we visited he used to say: 'Look! Another one has dropped dead. Why have they put me with all these old people who are all dropping dead?' He would be laughing his head off as he said it. We thought, *If only he knew that he is going to die himself.* It was black humour perhaps but my father found it very funny. He'd say: 'My God! They put a new one in and after three days he's gone!' But then he said: 'I'm getting fed up here – I feel as if I have to look after all these dying people.'

Then came another extraordinary surprise. One day out of the blue the doctor said: 'We are very sorry, we have diagnosed your father incorrectly. He does not have cancer, he is suffering from

TB – he can go home.' Everyone was astonished, but so pleased by this reprieve that we did nothing about this terrible medical mistake. But now, eleven years later, he became ill again, and this time he genuinely did have cancer. And this time he did not tell us. He only admitted the truth to our friend Marian, but he swore her to secrecy. And I am sure Esme, his lady friend, also knew about it. He did not want the family distressed so I suppose he played the joke on us in reverse.

We thought he was OK. He used to come to our house quite regularly when Sacha was five and Christian was four, and he would often have dinner with us. I remember one particular evening he came and he would not eat, though it was his favourite food, mussels. I knew he loved them and I thought this was very unusual. With hindsight I should have known that he was really ill but of course you don't think of it at the time.

He went into hospital, but we thought it was just more treatment for the TB. All of a sudden we got a phone call in the middle of the night to tell us that he had died. We were so shocked. Marian did the right thing for him but we all had things we would have said to my father, had we known how ill he was. We had no idea he was seriously ill – I think the fact that we did not know he had cancer made it more of a shock. In any case we were reeling, and not at all sure how to react. Unfortunately because he died so close to Christmas we could not have the funeral until the New Year. The salons were fully booked and we were really busy; every single one of us was completely booked up and so we took the decision to do what we thought my father would have wanted us to do: to carry on as normal and not let anyone down. So we delayed the funeral.

My father's death was extremely tragic and we all missed him very much. An extravagant character who brightened every room he entered, he had been there all our lives and it was shocking to realise he was all of a sudden no longer with us.

There was a strange footnote to my father's death that Pauline remembers best:

Two days after Toni's dad died, while we were still all in shock, I heard the noise of a door closing. I got up to go downstairs and as I was going out of the bedroom door, I met Sacha, coming out of her room. She was only six and she said, 'Mummy, Mummy, someone's in the other bedroom!' There was the presence of someone else in the house, but it was not frightening. Toni woke and I said, 'We don't have to worry. It's just your dad coming back to say goodbye.' And that is still exactly who I believe it was. We had visits from Toni's mum as well – it was a very happy house.

CHAPTER SEVEN

ADVENTURES OVERSEAS

T he death of my father on 18 December 1976 was a devastating blow to all of us and I certainly felt the loss very deeply indeed. I was all too aware that I was now the senior member of the family. Even though I had been running the family business for some years, the burden of responsibility seemed to weigh a little heavier, but in the whirlwind of work that surrounded me and my brothers there was never much time for worrying about anything for too long.

For two or three years the business had been exploding with activity. In 1974, we produced the first book to showcase our skills and it proved to be a huge success. We packed it full of photographs and the reaction was absolutely amazing. With books, photos, videos and the seminars, the Toni & Guy brand was fast becoming the hottest ticket in town. We were young and Italian and confident about our abilities as hairdressers to compete with the very best. It was a great time for all of us. Everything happened so fast and you could feel and see how proud my father was of his five sons' success. For me it was one of the most satisfying and rewarding times of my life.

And almost every day, in those too short years before he died, 'Pop' used to come to Davies Street. Always he would be immaculately dressed, in a smart suit with a white carnation in his buttonhole. He was a great character who never lost the ability to surprise me. I remember the day he gave me no choice with a sudden ultimatum that unless I arranged for a Gaggia coffee machine to be installed in Davies Street he would not come in any more. So I promptly ordered one.

A young man by the name of Luigi Guarneiri, who was at the time working for the then coffee wholesalers Costa, did a great job of installing the machine. He was a real expert and I have to say that after that my father would come into the salon and offer every client an espresso or a cappuccino. Then he would take great delight in personally making it for them. He loved doing it because most of all he loved providing good customer service – he knew it was part of the essential experience that helped to bring customers back to our salon. We served all sorts of coffees in the salon. We even used to do toasted sandwiches and other sorts of food as we became busier.

Occasionally the Italian Ambassador would pop in for an espresso on his way to the Embassy, which was situated along our street. In those days there were hardly any genuine coffee bars in London. I have no doubt that this must have encouraged the Costa brothers to open a coffee shop. That led to a chain and after that they definitely hit the jackpot when some years later they sold the business to Whitbread for a real fortune.

ADVENTURES OVERSEAS

★ ★ ★

Our first book was simply called *Hair:Toni & Guy* and was launched at our first show in 1974 at the Lancaster Hotel in London. Bruno, Anthony, Guy and myself were on stage and I remember so clearly there was no proper stand and at the front of the theatre there was my wife Pauline selling the first book herself and making friends with all the hairdressers. Our debut publication featured a photograph of my father in hairdressing action. It was a promising start and it gave a lift to us all to see our work in print.

Then we produced *Alta Moda* in 1978, which also did well, but our biggest success came the following year with the third book, *One Step Beyond*. It sold more than 30,000 copies very quickly indeed. I was extremely excited because we were breaking new ground. Vidal Sassoon had done well in the years before and he must never be forgotten for what he achieved, but our publications really were something new. With our tapes also on the market I knew some people thought that we might be making a mistake in showing so much of our work in such detail. People sometimes used to ask me if it was really at all wise to be so revealing of our skills and techniques. Many friends warned that we were in real danger of suffering commercially by giving away all our secrets so publicly.

To answer these questions and warnings I would tell a simple story to try to explain our confidence in opening up our salons and sharing our ideas. I told anyone who raised these concerns an old story about a certain Italian hairdresser who had learned a new haircut, which proved very popular. He had two or three apprentices, which was the way in those days, and he was afraid these apprentices would learn his technique, copy his style and take his clients away from him. So whenever he did a haircut he kept his hand in front of the client's hair to ensure his apprentices could not see what he was doing as he was cutting.

An excellent hairdresser, he had a tremendous amount of success with his style and lots of clients went to him. The danger with that was that he became so concerned with keeping his haircut to himself that he continued to do exactly the same thing over and over again. So when he reached five years down the line he found to his horror that styles had developed and moved on and become more popular, while he was still doing the same outdated thing. I pointed out to those who questioned our open policy that I didn't believe in that old hairdresser's philosophy; this particular Italian had become stuck in a time warp and I never wanted that for us. Most people seemed to get my message.

Our philosophy was and is that we create a new collection of styles and techniques and we show it to everybody as openly as possible and sell it through books and magazines. We then go on and create new styles, which are the next level so we can't ever just hide behind one style. People want new ideas and new styles all the time therefore that's what we gave them, and that's still what we give them today. All the time you have to progress and move on.

That was the philosophy of all of us. I can't claim individual credit – my brothers agreed wholeheartedly with me. This was just something that we all felt and believed in. We had total confidence in our ability to grow and develop and to keep coming up with new and popular styles. Although there is no denying there were plenty of arguments, about pretty much every subject under the sun, we agreed on far more than we disagreed about. And we all agreed on this maxim: if you stick with the same thing forever you get stuck in a rut, which can be good for a while but eventually leads you nowhere.

Pauline shrewdly observed how well we brothers worked together:

Toni and Guy were fantastic together. They were a brilliant combination because they were so different and they had completely different roles to play – that's why it worked so well. Guy was happy to leave all the business side to Toni, which was wise because Toni was always very careful. He has always believed in making money before spending it. Sometimes the brothers were inclined to do it the other way round. Guy was a brilliant hairdresser. Toni was more technical while Guy was very artistic; Toni was slower and very precise. The two of them were always very close. When Bruno and Anthony came into the business there was money there, that Toni and Guy had worked very hard to make, which enabled them to do their shows and photography.

Our first foray abroad came in 1975 when Guy was invited by a group of hairdressers to hold a seminar in Detroit, the centre of the then booming American motor industry. He accepted, and it was a huge success. In the United States he was treated like a king. He went over there not knowing quite what to expect and came back with a suitcase stuffed with money. Guy's outgoing personality was very popular – they loved his larger-than-life hairdressing style. I don't think they had seen anyone quite like him before. It was a brilliant experience for him. He said: 'Oh my God! Look at all these dollars! People went crazy to see me working – this is the way we've got to go.'

This led to us attending the huge international hairdressing exhibition at the New York Coliseum for the first time. It was another amazing experience. Doing shows up there on stage was something special – the audiences just loved us. Somehow we managed to make hairdressing look glamorous and exciting. We were all passionate about our work and that seemed to register with our audiences. Of course Anthony and Bruno, being younger, were perhaps the stars, but Guy was always a great hairdresser. I was the shyest and least showy of the brothers, but I still enjoyed my moments up there on stage. The audience reaction was fantastic, people even said we were like the Beatles! And that's just how it felt.

We used to sell our books and videos at the Coliseum exhibition and it was a wonderful event. I have to thank Freddie Laker for setting up his trail-blazing Skytrain, which was a great help to us when we wanted to fly across the Atlantic as cheaply as possible (always one of my main concerns – even when real success arrived, I was always very careful to do the best deal possible).

When we were in America we needed people to help on the stand and the local guys were charging $200 a day. That seemed much too high a price so I recruited Joy, one of our receptionists from London, to come over and help out. She was a beautiful girl, who was always very enthusiastic. I asked her if she would like to come to New York, stay in a top hotel and help out on the stand. She beamed at me and said: 'That would be my dream come true.' I had to admit that we were all sharing a couple of rooms in the hotel and she said: 'I don't mind sleeping on the floor if I'm going to New York!' I think I paid her £50 for her flight and she was absolutely brilliant at the job.

Joy was a very attractive blonde and the Americans simply

adored her. When she was on the stand there was always a queue of about fifty people waiting to hear her English accent. She sold lots of tapes and books and just about every sale was concluded with an invitation out to dinner. I would always step in and insist that she was staying in with me! And another time Ann, a Swedish receptionist who had different qualities, was even more valuable to me when I was organising a show in Stockholm.

She too was an extremely attractive blonde who was very persuasive with clients, intelligent and bright enough to keep quiet about her language skills. My Swedish clients asked me what price I was going to charge for the show and, guided by the British market, I decided the price should be around £5,000. But, fortunately for me, Ann had heard them talking together in Swedish and she quietly told me that they would be perfectly happy to pay a price of £12,000! So I made a much more handsome profit without too much effort.

★   ★   ★

In the early seventies London was the centre of education and students came from all over the world, including many from Japan. They introduced me to Japanese hairdressing scissors, which were much sharper than the ones we used in Europe. As soon as I started to try out some of the Japanese scissors, I realised they gave a hairdresser a very great advantage, particularly when it came to slide cutting and precision cutting. These Japanese scissors were the first ones I had come across that were so very, very sharp. They were much better than the French steel ones we had been using, which always needed sharpening after you had done a dozen haircuts otherwise your fingers would start really hurting.

Working with these Japanese scissors was like using a razor and they kept sharper for much longer, which enabled you to cut so many more people's hair. Later they even enabled our Toni & Guy skilled hairdressers to create and perfect new techniques such as intercutting and slice cutting, which was not possible with conventional scissors. I was at one of our exhibitions at the New York Coliseum, where I met Christopher Brooker, then head artistic director of Sassoon and a very famous hairdresser. I gave him a pair of Yasaka Japanese scissors. He used them extensively at the Sassoon Academy with all of his students and afterwards hundreds of them would come to Davies Street to purchase the scissors.

I realised this could become a very good investment for me because everyone wanted to buy these scissors and there was great potential for selling them all over the world so I set out to try to get the exclusive rights to them. I asked a Japanese student to introduce me to the manufacturer so that I could get world distribution because I thought if I could control the international sales I could sell thousands and thousands of these scissors all over the world. Unfortunately his English was a little bit weak and he introduced me, not to the manufacturer, but to the distributor, who did indeed give me exclusivity.

I started selling the scissors and they quickly proved remarkably popular, but very soon afterwards, I saw some Japanese scissors for sale in a shop that I knew I had not supplied. Even more disturbingly I discovered that wholesalers were selling them. I couldn't understand what on earth was going on so I telephoned the company in Japan and discovered to my horror that the company with whom I had done the deal was a distributor not the manufacturer. They had only given me my much-prized exclusivity to the scissors that they were selling. But clearly lots of other deals were in place with the manufacturer.

At one of our shows in London a rival hairdressing team came to one of our seminars (where Anthony was showing the twisted plait and weaving, which we were very strong with at the time) and we introduced them to our new Yasaka scissors. On my next visit to the New York Coliseum, I came upon this same hairdressing team showing these new techniques as their own and also using the latest Japanese scissors. The directors had cleverly gone to Japan themselves, found the real manufacturer and did a deal to sell the scissors in the United States. They made a fortune.

The experience taught me a lesson that I will never forget – don't make assumptions about who you are making deals with. I now also know that you learn much more from setbacks than from your successes. Throughout my life in business I have had many problems and difficulties and I believe they have taught me a great deal.

★   ★   ★

And I have certainly learned that business problems pale into the background when any sort of trouble affects my family. There was a heart-breaking tragedy on the home front that led to us leaving our much-loved home in Streatham. Our young Swedish au pair, who helped look after Sacha and Christian, was assaulted just outside our house. It was a terrible incident. She was a lovely young girl, who was kind as well as beautiful, and she was very happy living with us and being part of our family. Already she had asked Pauline if she could carry on living with us after the children grew older when she had finished being an au pair. She was hoping to get an office job in London for she just loved being in the city.

Then one night she came home at about 10 o'clock and everything changed. She told us that a man in a van had stopped and asked her the way. She went over to tell him and suddenly he grabbed and dragged her between two houses and raped her. It was an awful ordeal for this young girl, incredibly traumatic for her. It was a brutal, horrific attack and the police were not very supportive or sympathetic. This was 1977 and the investigation was not handled nearly as sensitively as it would be today.

She was absolutely devastated by the experience. Pauline and I thought the best thing would be for her to go back to Sweden so she could be with her mother; we thought her mum would be the one person who could help her. Unfortunately when she got home she discovered that her mother was more interested in her new boyfriend. The girl went to her room and stayed there for twenty-four hours. The next thing anyone knew was that she had committed suicide. It was a tremendous shock and it helped make up our minds to move further out. For us this was another turning point because it was by no means the only incident of this kind. The character of the neighbourhood was changing dramatically as more and more people from overseas arrived. Streatham was becoming quite rough and unsafe so we decided to look for a new home out in Surrey.

This was the time I always think that my faithful but forever cautious Mr Feak cost me a couple of a million pounds! We put our house on the market for £45,000. This was a healthy profit but we had made many improvements and by now it was 1978, a time when house prices were rocketing, as I was to learn to my considerable cost. Pauline found a lovely house in Burwood Park in Weybridge that she fell in love with. It was a veritable mansion – much bigger than the Streatham house and in a better area; another world from Streatham. It was priced at £72,000 and I thought to myself, *I've got to have that house. It's unbelievable!*

I turned to Mr Feak and said to him: 'We've got to get this house!' But he was unconvinced. I was sure I could squeeze a £30,000 mortgage but he warned darkly: 'Don't do it. It's too much commitment and it's too risky.' At first I refused to take no for an answer and almost pleaded with him to help me. This house was really special and, much more importantly, my wife had set her heart on it. But Mr Feak was adamant and very cautious. He said: 'I could help you, but I won't. It's too much.' So I took his advice and as a result I lost the house my wife and I had fallen in love with.

House prices were rising very fast at that time and six months later someone offered me £56,000 for the Abbotswood Road property. We still wanted to move and Pauline said: 'Now we can go and buy another one the same as the one we lost.' I thought we would probably have a chance to buy a similar house this time because I had saved up more money and would have the extra £11,000 from the sale of our house. I went back to the estate agent and explained that I wanted to buy a house just like the one I had sadly lost and now I had more money to pay for it. He said: 'I have some slightly bad news for you, Mr Mascolo. It will now cost you a minimum of £150,000 to £180,000 for the same type of house because prices of this type of property have more than doubled in six months!' So that was the end of my chances of getting my wife's dream house at that time. And I realised then that you should always go with your instinct and make your own decision. This is the philosophy that has helped me for many years since; I have been able to grow the Toni & Guy empire by backing my own decision whenever it has conflicted with the view of the experts.

Later on we went to a new development in Ashcroft Park, Cobham. They were building new houses there so we put our name down and eventually bought a house on the estate. It was a lovely area and a fantastic place, with very friendly neighbours from the United States, Holland, Italy and other parts of the world, but the house was possibly a quarter of the size of the one I had lost six months previously and the price was £80,000. Everything was miniature compared to the other house but nevertheless that was what it was and we bought it. We spent three lovely years in this house and our youngest child Pierre was born there. My wife continued looking for something bigger and soon she fell in love with a house in Wrens Hill, Oxshott. It had an amazing view; you could see right across the countryside to Dorking from the house. On a new estate built by a Mr North, it was called North Court Park Estate. However, the house my wife fell in love with actually belonged to the builder, Mr North, and he was not interested in selling.

Then one day in 1982 Pauline was shopping in Epsom when she saw the house was up for sale and she came home extremely excited. She could not believe it, so we made enquiries to see if we could buy it. We agreed a price and quickly got in touch with the solicitors to purchase the house and make our dream come true. We made money on our house and did very well, it sold for £120,000, and the other house was £140,000. The solicitor went straight to London to meet the other owner's solicitor to exchange on the other property.

I was cutting hair in Davies Street when I got a shocking call from my solicitor. He was very embarrassed and he admitted that sometimes he was ashamed of the actions of some members of his own profession. Evidently, at the very last minute before contracts were exchanged the vendor's solicitor had asked for another £5,000 on behalf of the vendor or the deal was off. It was an awful lot of money in those days but fortunately for us my brother Guy had some money because he had just sold his penthouse flat in Bournemouth. Without a moment's hesitation Guy said: 'I'll give you the £5,000 and then you can pay me back when you can.' It was very generous of him and I've never forgotten it.

So we went ahead and bought it. Nevertheless, although this house was definitely a move up in the world, it was obvious that it wasn't nearly as grand and impressive as the one we had originally lost. That's why I've always thought that Mr Feak's cautiousness cost me a fortune.

This was perhaps one of the toughest times of my life. My wife was not at all well, work was extremely demanding and I had to travel abroad more and more, which was very hard on Pauline. She recalls:

I understood that Toni needed to travel a lot for the business and I always told the children that it was because Daddy loved us so much that he was far away, working hard to provide for us. It was not easy but sometimes we just had to love him from a distance. That was the truth so I never complained. But it was hard on Toni and it was hard on me as well. He was just so determined to make the family business a success and although the other brothers played different parts, I believe it was mainly down to Toni being so driven and working so hard that success eventually arrived.

Money was not really the great driving force for either of

us. I did not marry a rich man and we were every bit as happy in our early days when we had nothing as ever we were later on when the business did well. I had always wanted a really big family; four or five children at least. Unfortunately I was not well for six or seven years after having Christian. Even when we could afford help I almost always looked after the two youngest myself. They were always with me, I could never let them out of my sight. I was always frightened something would happen to them. The memory of Toni losing his mum was always there.

The glandular fever virus that was found in my blood remained there in spite of all the efforts of doctors. They couldn't get rid of it and it is still there today. It still sometimes makes me very weak, I'm afraid. In our early days as a family it was very hard for Toni because I know that he worried an awful lot about me on top of all his business problems.

Although we both really wanted to have more children after Christian was born, it took me six years to get pregnant again. Tragically we lost that baby. We were both desperately sad. Then it took me another two years to fall pregnant again, this time with a second son we called Pierre. He was born just after we had moved to a new house in Cobham. So each of our three children were born into different homes.

The Davies Street salon was bursting at the seams with activity. I was delighted that so many clients from Clapham had followed us up to Davies Street to have their hair done. We had always been very busy in Clapham but in Davies Street, with all of us in action, it was a real hive of activity. The days when we had desperately struggled to get our styles into print were long gone, now it was not simply the free magazines like *Ms London* and *Girl About Town* who were featuring our photographs. We had *Harpers & Queen* keen to feature a spread on 'The Chunky Look', which was one of our many popular new creations. And the magazine of the trade, the highly respected *Hairdressers Journal*, was more than happy to publish a very positive article praising 'The Toni & Guy philosophy'.

One of Anthony's most eye-catching styles was the twisted plait, which quickly attracted a lot of attention. It was featured at many of our seminars and involved a complex technique, which was not at all easy to master. One particular group of Americans, who had flown over especially for a Toni & Guy course, were treated to an insight into how exactly to perfect a twisted plait by a rather junior member of the Mascolo family – I think Sacha was eight years old when she came up to Davies Street with her mum. Even as a child she always loved the busy atmosphere of the salon and that day she quickly disappeared into the bustling maze.

I was heavily involved with the business of the day and it was not until a while later that I found time to go back downstairs in search of her. When I walked into the seminar room I was shocked and embarrassed to find her at the centre of all our hairdressing students, happily holding forth to a rapt audience. Here was this eight-year-old girl showing several Americans how to do these twisted plaits! I said: 'I'm really sorry.' These Americans were paying a lot of money to receive our help and tuition, they could hardly have expected to be lectured by a young child. I tried to apologise that they were 'being annoyed' by my young daughter.

'Being *annoyed*?' came the reply. 'Your daughter has been here for twenty minutes and we have learned more in that time than we have in the whole week. She is fantastic! Under no circumstances are you going to take her away from us.'

You know what happens – children can explain things very simply.

They do it so naturally. She was just showing them, and saying, 'You put your fingers like that and you twist the hair around', so they could understand, and they would not let her go. I will never forget the scene— they just thought my daughter was so wonderful and of course like any proud father, deep down I agreed. They wanted to keep her there all day, but I managed to drag Sacha away after a couple of hours. She was really enjoying herself.

Sacha recalls:

I always loved visiting the salon with my dad. We've always been incredibly close and I loved to spend time with him whenever I got the chance. The salon in Davies Street was a wonderful place. Right from as far back as I can remember I loved everything about the people and the atmosphere. I loved hairdressing from being very young and I could do the twisted plaits and I loved showing people. That time I was just trying to be helpful, I didn't realise I was lecturing real students!

My dad was away a lot when I was younger because in the early days he had nothing. The first house I remember was in Abbotswood Road, Streatham and it was very ordinary. I lived there until I was eight and then we moved to Surrey. My dad used to go to Japan a lot when I was younger and when he came back he had this great enthusiasm about the Japanese. He always used to say how amazing they were at business, and this was just when Japanese technology was really booming. My dad used to bring me back these lovely Japanese dolls and I had this real thing about Japan as well.

★　★　★

Although we were very busy in the salons I was travelling the world more and more as I became convinced that ours was a business with enormous international potential. Even so I was pretty astonished by the contents of a telephone call out of the blue from Dax Uinagi, the English-speaking representative of a giant Japanese corporation run by Koichi Takigawa. I was really busy with clients in the salon, but Dax was a nice guy and the Takigawa Company was then the twenty-sixth largest company on the Japanese stock market, so I took the call. The huge business sold a wide range of products including all hairdressing equipment from scissors to mirrors and furniture.

'Mr Takigawa would like you to come to our exhibition in Japan next week,' said Dax. That seemed completely out of the question and I said: 'Thank you very much. That is very kind of you, but I'm fully booked and very busy in the salon.' But Dax was very persistent. He explained that it was a great honour to receive this sort of invitation from Mr Takigawa, and he added that if I came to Japan and brought with me the original U-matic master tapes from our first basic beginners' step-by-step educational videotapes, then Mr Takigawa would be very interested in purchasing them.

The tapes were all now well out of date and completely worthless to me. Our hairdressing had moved on and developed a great deal since they were made and the quality was less than perfect. There were fourteen of them gathering dust in an archive and already we had made plans to produce new ones, so I couldn't see they had any further value to the company. Nevertheless Mr Takigawa said he would pay us £2,000 for each one if I brought them with me to Japan. He obviously wanted me to be present at his exhibition; he must have thought my presence would be valuable to him. I was astonished – this was a serious sum of money. In those days £28,000 would have bought a nice flat in Mayfair.

Dax said: 'Bring the tapes to Japan and we'll give you the money.' I said I would be there as soon as I could get a flight. 'We can arrange that,' he told me. He sent me a ticket and two days later I went to Japan. I had never been there before and in those days it was quite a journey. I flew from London to Dubai and then on to Bangkok, Hong Kong, Taipei, and eventually into Tokyo. It was a very long haul, a real adventure. I arrived at Mr Takigawa's exhibition and was instantly amazed by the colossal scale of the operation.

The event was staged at a huge place that must have been ten times the size of Earls Court – it was enormous! There were more than 200 people wearing the Takigawa shirt and running the show. Evidently Mr Takigawa's enterprise was involved with more than 1,000 manufacturing companies and the exhibition attracted over 4,000 different hairdressing wholesalers, who sold just about anything you could imagine. Occasionally there was an announcement over the loudspeaker and everyone went quiet and then there would be lots of wild cheering. I was told that this meant that someone had reached his sales target. As we were walking through the exhibition Mr Takigawa stopped one of his employees and asked him to do a task but the employee kept bowing and bowing, and thanking him continuously. He was so pleased to have been chosen; so proud.

I thought of that on my return to London when I asked a salon assistant to make me a cup of coffee. She didn't bow to me or even nod, come to that. She barely bothered to look in my direction and just said: 'Can't Jackie do it? I am going to lunch in a minute.' Clearly, we had a lot to learn from the Japanese!

As the exhibition neared its conclusion I learned they had taken some $385 million. *Wow, that's a lot of money!* I thought. Then eight policemen came in with a huge amount of cash. When Mr

Takigawa paid the discount to the distributors who placed the orders he preferred to hand it over in advance, in cash. I watched, open-mouthed, as millions of dollars in cash changed hands before my very eyes. When his distributors had made orders up to $100,000 they received 20 per cent in advance in cash on signing the order that would be paid for a month later. Later I told people in Europe and America about this instant reward system and they all said we should try it in our business. By then I had learned a little more about the Japanese way of life and so I had my answer ready. I always said: 'No, because if these guys don't pay the invoice after they have taken the discount they are so honourable and so proud in some cases they would even commit suicide. You lot would probably just disappear!'

I seemed to hit it off very well with Mr Takigawa. I realised that the reason he got me there was because I was a famous hairdresser from London and he just wanted to be with me. He took me to the best places in Tokyo – to the top clubs, restaurants and shows – and he was at all times a very generous host. I have never seen anyone give so much money away! He was forever tipping people – anybody who bowed to him, or served him with a cup of coffee or did anything for him, he would give the equivalent of a £50 note. He sprayed money around like confetti,– I had never seen so much wealth.

Eventually we came to my money. He asked me how I wanted to be paid. I said boldly: 'Cash would be nice.' I was naïve, but I didn't know what else to say after what I had just witnessed. Mr Takigawa gave me a case with the Japanese money in it. In those days £1 was worth 800 yen; the highest note was 10,000 yen. There were masses of notes, I felt as if I had raided a bank.

I didn't know anything about currency transfers in those days. Were you allowed to take the money out of the country? I had no idea what the law said, but I had an invoice and I had the money. When I got to the airport my case went through the machine without incident. I retraced my tortuous journey, travelling through Taipei, which made Japan seem luxurious in comparison, through Hong Kong to Bangkok. I was faced with an 18-hour stop in the capital of Thailand so I decided I would come out of the airport for a while and have a look round the city. Then I thought again. Suddenly I felt a little uneasy wandering round an unfamiliar city carrying a huge sum of money with me. I knew that with the amount of cash in that case you could have lived like a millionaire in Thailand for the rest of your life. And it would have been very difficult to go back in through customs once you came out of the airport. Thank God I decided not to leave the airport, otherwise I think there is a good chance that I would not be here today.

I stayed inside in the building with the other in-transit passengers and when I was ready to board the plane for London, I went through security. The security man asked me to open the case. I was annoyed and said: 'Why? I am in transit.' But he insisted. Reluctantly, I opened the case and he saw all the money and immediately started yelling: 'Money, Money, Money!' at the top of his voice. 'Shut up!' I said, 'What's it got to do with you what I have in the case? I am in transit!' I was thinking to myself that there are lots of tall, big passengers around me and it wouldn't be very wise to let them know that I had all of this money in my case. Bizarrely, the security man quickly calmed down and allowed me through to board the plane. It was a nasty scare but I thought my problems were over as I settled into my seat. I was just beginning to relax and was sitting back, thinking, *Thank goodness for that*, but just as I was in the process of closing my eyes for a relaxing snooze I heard a couple of ominous clicks.

My eyes flicked open and I was terrified to see two machine guns pointing directly at me on both sides of my head: two uniformed men with guns. I was shocked at first and then terrified, and I shouted: 'What do you want?' And they said: 'You carrying money!' So I said, still quite aggressively, that I was in transit from Japan. I explained I had done a business deal and I had sold some educational hairdressing videotapes to the Takigawa Company. 'It's really got nothing to do with you guys in Thailand,' I said, and I then showed them the invoice. They looked at it, thought about it a little, and then mercifully their attitudes seemed to change. The guy in charge said abruptly: 'OK,' and they turned away and got off the plane.

It was an unnerving experience but once the plane had taken off and I was convinced it was all over, I gradually relaxed in my seat and started feeling very proud of myself. I had lots of satisfaction and felt very joyful over what I had achieved and all the money I had made in such a short period. When I got home I couldn't wait to show my wife all the cash and instantly she said: 'Good, we can buy a lot of things with all that cash, let's keep it!' Of course I wanted to show my brothers and everyone in the company what I had done and I couldn't wait to get the lot of it into the bank. At the time it was the best deal of my life. It was my first export, and it was done alone.

That trip was the first of very many journeys to Japan. I was always looking for new ways in which to develop our business and the Japanese in those days were on the crest of a profit-making wave. Mr Takigawa soon asked me to go to Japan for a second time. There was another exhibition, but this time it was mainly for wholesalers. He gave them vouchers and the more vouchers they gave to the hairdressers, the more discount the wholesalers received. So when the hairdresser went to spend money they didn't use money, they used the credit vouchers from the wholesaler. So, of course, the hairdressers were even keener to buy as much as possible, which they wouldn't have bought if they had used cash. It was a simple but cleverly constructed system and, as far as I could see, it worked brilliantly.

Mr Koichi Takigawa was one of the most powerful businessmen in Japan. He might have left school at ten, but he never stopped learning and what an amazing brain he had. That's why I always say I learned a lot from the Japanese. My trips were a great success. I learned a lot about the Japanese people as well. First and foremost, they are a very, very proud race. They feel superior to everyone else, a little bit like the Germans. When you go into negotiations with people from other parts of the world, I learned early on, it is often very different. The Israelis bargain very hard and so do the Italians, though as you might expect with a little more style. Commerce started with the Chinese and you can always make a deal with them. The Anglo-Saxons and the Germans are a little bit straighter: if there is a deal to be done you can go directly to it – they are quite straightforward. The Japanese are different.

We had produced our first books on hairdressing and I was keen to learn the skills of international negotiating pretty quickly. When it came to the Chinese, if you wanted to sell, say, 100 books for £7 each then you might say if you buy 1,000, they will be £6 each, and if you buy 5,000, the unit price will be £5. The Chinese would offer you £4.50 for 5,000 and make a deal. The Japanese would just say: 'No, it's too expensive.' You have to offer them a good deal up front if you want their interest in the first place. A friendly Japanese buyer explained it to me: 'We want to buy, but we don't want to bargain. We are not like the Chinese – just give us the best price.'

But even that was fraught with pitfalls. It cost about £3.50 a copy to produce the book in those days, so I thought, *I'll tell him the price is £4.50 and make £1 a copy.* He wanted 5,000 books so I said it would be £4.50 a copy. Then he said he would like to buy 10,000, so I thought in that case it would be safe to say £4 a copy. So I would still make £5,000. But then he said £3.50. I said: 'No, you told me the best price, I can't do it at £3.50. That's what it costs me.' So I lost the deal. Why? Because the Japanese are very proud, they must always have the last word so you need to be a little bit over if you want to do a deal.

I learned another important lesson: the Japanese really do always think they are superior. They are humble and gentle on the surface but underneath they are totally convinced they are better than you in every way. On another very difficult deal I was close to reaching an agreement, but then I lost my temper because I'd had enough. The haggling had gone on for three weeks and eventually I just ran out of patience and said that I didn't want to do the deal any more. I said: 'Can I tell you something. I know deep in my heart that you are messing around here because you think you are superior and that you want your own way and nothing else. You ought to know I come from the dynasty that built the Roman Empire and I feel superior to you. Let's cut the bullshit and make a deal.' And, surprise, surprise, we made a deal. In the end I felt very proud of myself because I was beginning to think I had lost this one.

★   ★   ★

I was very proud of our first books and I really wanted to sell them in the biggest market in the world, the United States of America. Unfortunately I had no real contacts until I took matters into my own hands and attended a hairdressing exhibition at the New

York Coliseum, one of the biggest in the USA, with the official English party. I visited one of the stands that seemed to specialise in selling books. The owner wasn't there but a member of staff told me that the person I needed to speak to was a gentleman called Joe Chiriello. Instantly I pricked up my ears because Chiriello is a Neapolitan name. I left one of our books with the staff member and told her that I would be in the Barbizon Plaza in case Mr Chiriello was interested in the distribution for America.

Bruno and I had travelled with the *Hairdressers Journal*, which was then edited by Mr Norman Bloomfield. He brought a lot of different hairdressers together and he helped to organise everything. When I got back to the hotel I received a phone call from Joe Chiriello. He was very excited, saying he was staying at the same hotel as me, that he wanted to take me out for dinner and he might be interested in our book. I explained that I would be accompanied by my brother Bruno and a friend, who was called Martin.

Back then I was a bit nervous and I had met Martin on my way to New York for the first time. A fiery guy with bright red hair, he had really penetrating eyes and he seemed like a nice guy. He was asking me all about Toni & Guy and he clearly seemed to love our company. An experienced wholesaler with a reputation for being a bit of a wheeler and dealer, he was a well-known figure. I thought it might be wise to bring him along because he would perhaps be able to give me some support and help negotiate as he had a lot of experience. Martin quickly accepted the invitation and said he was ready for the challenge and happy to advise me. We arranged to meet at eight, but Joe Chiriello didn't turn up.

After a lengthy wait and some confused phone calls it turned out he was at the wrong hotel! He was in the Plaza, not the Barbizon Plaza, but eventually we managed to sort it out and meet for dinner, although by that time it was getting quite late. He insisted on taking us to one of the top restaurants in New York. Joe Chiriello was from Chicago. He told us he was Al Capone's grandson. He was very upfront and in our faces, acting like a small-time gangster from the old days, and he kept mentioning his famous grandfather and how powerful the relationship had made him.

We went to this classy restaurant and the waiter came and brought bread and water and welcomed us; we had a chat and a few minutes later he arrived with the menu. And Joe turned to the waiter arrogantly and said, 'What's that?' The waiter said: 'This is the menu, sir, for you to choose.' Joe Chiriello shouted: 'I don't need any menus! I am Joe Chiriello from Chicago and these are my guests and I just want you to bring the best food and drink you've got for my friends.' We were all totally shocked – it was like being in some kind of a gangster scene in one of those Hollywood films. Nevertheless I suppose we were very excited to be part of that crazy scene and started enjoying the best treatment and the best food that this waiter could bring us. We were, after all, Joe Chiriello's guests. Although I had started out just trying to sell my books to this chap, his behaviour and personality were starting to take everything over.

To make the situation even more crazy, out of the blue my new associate Martin jumped out of his chair and went over to the table next to us to greet this beautiful woman, who just happened to be Margaret Trudeau, wife of the then Prime Minister of Canada. Thanks to her colourful dalliances with rock stars and politicians, which were all over the newspapers, she was quite a well-known personality in those days. She was accompanied by a tall and sophisticated and very classy-looking gentleman, who looked very distinguished – he gave me the impression he was either a politician or a film producer.

To my surprise I overheard Martin introduce himself to this glamorous celebrity as 'the manager of Toni & Guy, famous hairdressers from London'. I also heard him telling Mrs Trudeau that Toni Mascolo was at the next table and he would love to meet her. They had finished eating and to my astonishment they joined us for a drink, by which time Joe Chiriello was merrily smoking marihuana as well as drinking. This was clearly a night for surprises. I am proud to say that all through the sixties, I never ever smoked anything or took any drugs. To me it seemed like a complete waste of time and money. I was never remotely interested and I was very wary of any kind of drug.

Joe Chiriello, Bruno and Martin all joined the party and I was astonished to see that Margaret Trudeau was also quite relaxed about joining in. It was the end of the night and I think she was a bit tipsy. I sat back, absorbing the scene and the atmosphere, and I couldn't help thinking to myself, *Here I am, sitting here in New York City with this most glamorous, well-known lady, who is featured in every magazine and newspaper, and we are having such a good time!* It was a marvellous moment.

I also noticed that Margaret Trudeau and my brother Bruno seemed to be getting on very well and a few significant glances were exchanged between them. I think he had developed a soft spot for her. She was a very attractive lady so I couldn't blame him but Bruno was very shy and I don't think anything ever came of it. It was a strange and unforgettable evening. Best of all, Joe Chiriello ordered 5,000 books and so we sold our first copies in America.

Doing business in the United States was clearly going to be different.

CHAPTER EIGHT

'THE BEATLES OF HAIRDRESSING'

W e all knew America could be a very important part of our future but it was difficult for us to establish ourselves because we had no base or family there. We were making contacts but we were still dependent on the people we met who wanted to do business with us.

A year after meeting Joe Chiriello, at the next annual exhibition at the New York Coliseum, I met someone else who was also keen to work with us. Ken Mandel was a very outgoing American chap with a hairdressing salon near Dallas in Texas. It was very well run by his wife, who was herself an excellent and hard-working hairdresser. Ever-confident Ken thought of himself as much more of a businessman, though, and was full of ideas for deals. 'I would like you boys to come out and do a show in Dallas, Texas,' he said. 'They would love Toni & Guy and you don't realise how famous you are there.'

Stunned, I said: 'You mean Dallas, Texas… as in Cowboys and

Indians?' As a boy I had always loved playing Cowboys and Indians. Impressed by this approach, I thought, *We can't refuse this!* We discussed lots of different options of how this would happen and at first we were very impressed by Mandel. At the end of the day, as we were to learn later, he was only a small salon owner with a big dream, who thought we could make him lots of money.

He offered to pay all our expenses, including all flights and accommodation, and suggested we split the profits equally. He seemed very excited and equally sure that this venture would generate a big profit for all of us. I was enthusiastic: after all, it was not going to cost us anything and I would be able to spend time in the place of my childhood dreams.

We stayed in a huge luxury hotel called the Anatole – it was very famous at the time. In the middle of the hotel there was a square with grass and trees. It was like a lovely park, right in the hotel. It was such an unbelievable place and that was where we were going to do all our shows. We all had enormous suites as we took over the whole of the top floor and no expense was spared looking after us. Ken Mandel even had a girl outside our rooms cheerfully pouring champagne all day! The suites were luxurious as well as vast. We held our model castings there and it was a memorable experience – there were lots of beautiful women everywhere.

I've never seen so many stunning girls in one place at the same time. We did so many shows together, we had quite an act and quite a presence on the stage. And the reaction from American audiences was absolutely out of this world. Again, they said we were 'the Beatles of hairdressing' and they screamed and cheered so much I think they meant it too. Bruno, Guy, Anthony and I received a wonderful reception. The audiences really seemed to love us and of course we loved every minute of it. Who wouldn't?

We brought in so much money that at one point we had a suitcase full of dollars. It felt as if we four brothers were conquering America together. It seemed too good to be true, and in many ways it was. Although the amazing reception was real enough, the bill from the hotel was so enormous that in the end we never made a penny profit out of the whole exhilarating exercise. Ken Mandel had installed us in one of the most expensive hotels in America and that was where all the money went.

But in many ways it was still the best thing that ever happened to us. Money was not important (definitely not something you will hear me say very often!) – it was the whole amazing experience that taught us something. It was out of this world. The Americans just loved our style of hairdressing and it helped to convince me we had a business which would work worldwide.

Some of the models were so excited they were really keen to continue working with us and we obviously wanted to spend more time in the United States. We tried to find ways to make this possible so we decided to sell our videos, books and posters. Of course Mr Ken Mandel was happy to offer to open an office that he would run and deal with sales. The girls were ready to help us, but unfortunately we had no work permits or relevant visas. Naively, we hadn't even thought about the important paperwork – we relied on Mr Mandel, but he was not one of the brothers. He had a totally different attitude and was possibly a little bit too aggressive in a style that did not work too well with our beloved models. And although we sold lots of videos, books and posters, by the time all the expenses of rent, and wages for the girls and Mr Mandel had been paid, there was no profit again. I should have learned my lesson the first time. It was a great try but the only way it would have succeeded in America is if one of the brothers had moved there.

We lost most of the girls because while they wanted to work with us, they most certainly didn't want to work with Mr Mandel. They had only come to Dallas in the first place for a chance to work with us for very little money.

But they were fascinating times. Dallas in those days was like the Wild West. The oil came up out of the ground and it seemed as if everybody and his brother was coming to Dallas to get rich. It was a mad place – it was just unbelievable the money you could make. There were so many people with a lot of money to spend, far more than in Britain or anywhere else.

America was the place where it seemed that anyone with a five-year plan to become a millionaire could succeed. People really did get rich quick. That was the time when everything started to develop. I began to set my mind on expansion. Building was going on all over the place and thousands of young people were coming to live and work there. Waiters could make more than a hundred dollars a night just on tips! There was an amazing amount of growth in the next two years. I went over there several times during that time. It was growing so fast. I made a lot of contacts and it was a very interesting time. It was an enormous pity that I didn't have a visa and couldn't actually work there.

I first saw franchising in the United States, but it was very different from what we later created over here and all over the world. Franchising over there was simply someone getting a salon and then renting chairs and bringing in their own clients and taking 60 or 70 per cent of the money. Hairdressing in America was seen as much more of a job whereas in England we had helped to develop it as an art.

In America, it seemed you could never become truly accepted as an artist unless you specialised in something more obviously artistic like painting or sculpture. Hairdressing was considered much more commercial in America and I think that is why it would never create anyone nearly as artistic as the hairdressers we developed in Britain. What we created in the UK was very different. We designed new styles and specialised in colour and we were developing all the time. Always we were experimenting and changing in cutting and in fashion. There was specialisation in every aspect of hairdressing. We produced really new hairstyles that were different and we publicised them.

The American hairstylists came to our seminars, learned our styles and then went back and did the hair of many actresses and models in America. Whenever they appeared in magazines or on television it gave the impression that the styles were American, but they were English and in most cases they came from Toni & Guy. Sometimes this was frustrating, but we just had to accept it. The importance of America was the outlets it gave to us, which were to become very lucrative.

★   ★   ★

Back in the United Kingdom our salon in Davies Street just got busier and busier throughout the 1970s. Towards the end of the decade I was searching for more space, both for a second salon and for a base for a proper Toni & Guy Academy. Finding the right property is never easy, but I thought I had struck lucky when I talked to an old friend and long-established hairdresser called Harold Leyton. He had a son who wanted to train to be a hairdresser and I agreed to put Harold's son in our seminars and give him a free hairdressing education.

At that time Harold was running a salon in Wimpole Street. He had previously been involved in big business deals and he didn't seem very happy to be back behind the chair, feeling and now he clearly felt out of place. I had the idea I might be able to take over his salon in Wimpole Street. I told him that if he wanted to sell the place then I would be prepared to buy it and turn it into an academy. The idea seemed to appeal to him and we agreed I would pay £18,000 for his place. We shook hands and I was very happy with the deal, until a week or so later when he rang up and said some guy who wanted to open a chemist's had offered him £1,000 more. He tried to apologise and said: 'What can I do? A grand is a grand.' And he asked me: 'What would you have done in my place?' I said: 'I think you did the right thing for you, it's more profitable for you, what else can I say?'

In fact I was extremely upset and I felt very let down because I was really looking forward to opening our first academy and it would have been a great opportunity. When it happened I thought, *What would I have done if the positions of Harold and myself had been reversed?* Well, I would certainly not have been like him and gone back on our agreement. My word is my bond, and so it would have been had I been in his position. As it was I put it down as another lesson that I learned in business. Later on I met Harold on many different occasions at exhibitions and hairdressing shows and we were able to laugh together over the lost deal. After all, we were men of the world. So we lost out on Wimpole Street, but fortunately soon afterwards I found a much better place to be the home of our first proper academy.

I was looking at a building in St Christopher's Place and as soon as I went inside I knew it would be absolutely perfect for our school. It was ideal. I said to myself: 'God has been good to me.' Straight away I decided I would take it. The estate agent asked me if I was sure I didn't want to think about it. 'No, I'll have it now,' I told him. He said he had never heard of anything like that before, and had never experienced anyone making a decision so quickly without taking a little time to think about it. I explained that when you know something is good for you, you only take a second to make your mind up – and in all honesty I have been doing this ever since.

Often today when I am confronted with a franchisee who has all the abilities, the capital, talent and everything in place to make a great success of a franchise and a business and sometimes it doesn't go through and doesn't happen, then I later realise that they might have everything except that important little thing called courage. So that's why, when I think of something I really want, I go for it there and then. It's a way of working that has helped me to be the person that I am and to grow the business in the way I've done it. So I told the agent to come to Davies Street there and then and I would sign whatever needed to be signed.

Soon afterwards, we opened our first Toni & Guy school for hairdressers. We needed more and more trained hairdressers, so it was the next step in our growth. Toni & Guy St Christopher's Place went from strength to strength and became recognised as one of the best academies in the world, not only for the strong education it provided but also for its perfect location in the heart of London, which had a tremendous amount of atmosphere in those days.

Davies Street was bursting at the seams when we at last found our next salon. It was in Sloane Square and at the time operated by a very traditional hairdresser called Richard Conway. Something of a legend at the time, he had been at the heart of the hairdressing world for many years. He ran the Ginger Group and also had another salon round the corner on Lower Sloane Street, as well as many other salons in London. Richard used the Sloane Square salon as a coffee bar and a hairdressing salon. I wasn't sure if it really mattered much to him any more as he had a great many other salons.

I had a meeting with him and I was very nervous and almost sure that I wasn't ever going to get this opportunity to take over his salon because there were so many other hairdressers interested in it. I tried to be as courteous and complimentary to him as I could and explained that I respected all his achievements. I told him that I had always looked up to him, but now we were the new boys in town and we needed more salons to grow into. It would be a tremendous help if he would sell his salon to us. He seemed uninterested, but then I tried to explain that we might be of some use to him and that we could share some of our education and help train some of his staff as we were very busy and well-known in central London. He seemed to react quite favourably to that idea and asked me to meet him again at his office. It was the first time I actually saw a hairdresser with his own office and PA. I think this PA must have worked for him all her life as she was probably in her late seventies, though she was still very sharp and on the ball in her knowledge of all his businesses.

To my astonishment Richard Conway seemed to take quite a liking to my humble approach and he said: 'Yes, I might sell it to you.' Eventually we made a deal that we would give a year of free education to anyone that he wanted to send to us as we turned the downstairs of the Sloane Square salon into an academy. I have to say this was probably the best deal of my life. Sloane Square is one of the most sought-after and prestigious locations in London. Our salon has always been very profitable and over the years we have had numerous famous hairdressers visiting us.

Richard never took up the offer of sending anyone in for education. He thought about it and realised it might not be a good idea so he asked for a credit instead of sending staff to be trained by us. He said that it might not have been in his interest or to his advantage but I politely said: 'That was part of my budget and a deal is a deal, sir.'

CHAPTER NINE

ROMAN INTERLUDE

I t's just under 900 miles from London to Rome as the crow flies, but suburban Clapham Park Road is a world away from stylish Via Frattina in the capital of Italy. Yet that was the switch we made in 1978 when the money from our original south London salon went to help fund an exciting expansion into Europe that took us back into our beloved home country. It should have been our happiest enterprise, but it didn't quite work out like that.

After the long hours I had worked in Clapham I had grown quite fond of Toni & Guy's humble first home, but I was still pleased to see it go. The wrangle with lazy John, the manager who turned our clients away because he couldn't be bothered to take care of them, had soured the place a little for me. But the decision to leave the salon was not mine in any case. After the Queen's Silver Jubilee celebrations in 1977 the local council decided to redevelop the area of Clapham where our shop stood and we were duly awarded some £14,000 in compensation. It might not sound much nowadays but back then it was quite a useful sum. We used the money, and some of our savings from the years since we set up the business, to open a new salon in Rome. We were always hoping one day to go back to our beloved Italy and have a Toni & Guy salon there. It was our dream, though I'm not sure we ever believed that it would become a reality, especially in Rome, the eternal city.

My brother Bruno was always the driving force behind the Rome project. He took charge of the opening of the salon. From the start he was extremely excited and highly motivated. Bruno was only eight years old when he left Italy and came to England and I think he felt it was part of his heritage to return to his homeland to run a hairdressing salon. He had an Italian friend called Maurizio Zangheri, who used to come to some of our seminars. Maurizio already had a very good salon of his own, just outside the centre of Rome on an expensive new development called EUR on the way to the airport. The residents there were mostly well-off professionals and middle-class Romans and already he had managed to build up a very busy and profitable business.

Maurizio was very keen to go into partnership with us to open a new salon on the famous Via Frattina. He absolutely idolised Bruno and the plan was that we would go in 50–50 with him. We got all our money together and sixteen years of carefully accumulated savings plus the council's compensation all went to set up the great new Rome venture. My wife Pauline was dead against the idea from the start, and of course with hindsight I know that I should have listened more carefully to her warnings. She is a wise and sensible woman. But unfortunately I allowed myself to be persuaded by Bruno's passionate enthusiasm and we went ahead with the project. It all started so well; we got ourselves the most amazing salon. It was twenty years ahead of anything anyone else had in Rome.

Bruno had already successfully worked with a very charismatic lady called Sonia Mellet and he wanted to involve her in the opening. She was a colourful Albanian princess, who was very well connected. We decided, Sonia and us four brothers, that we wanted to do something really amazing for the launch of our salon. We even chartered a plane to take all our VIP guests from London. We invited anyone that we felt could bring something special to the launch, including many journalists and press people, along with many of our most high-profile clients. Norman Broomfield, the editor of *Hairdressers Journal*, and many other important and influential people from the media world were flown over.

Sonia Mellet had been involved in many of our shows. Extremely beautiful, fashionable and supremely confident, she was very enthusiastic about going to Rome, and indeed it was where she was to meet the film directors who eventually helped to fulfil her dream of getting into movies. She added a touch of glamour and helped to bring in important guests, compiling a list that included the son of the former Italian President, Mr Giovanni Leone. There were many members of Italian high society, including countesses and even the famous actress Gina Lollobrigida, who later on helped us to do an amazing commercial, which was totally new and inventive, on Italian national TV. It was just an amazing time in our lives and we felt this was the start of something really, really big; we took Rome by storm.

The lavish opening was a great occasion and at first the Rome salon seemed to be going very well. The expensive opening appeared to have paid off and early bookings were very healthy. For six months everything went really well and it seemed our investment was a sound one. Maurizio looked up to my brother Bruno as if he was a little god. He said Bruno was his inspiration.

It was great for us to spend time in Italy. Our second son Pierre was born in 1979 and I was so happy we were able to have his christening in my home country. The christening was organised by a wonderful young Italian girl called Nilda. She was from Florence and had worked in England and then gone back to Rome to work. She was very friendly with my brother Guy. Nilda was remarkable! She arranged everything for Pierre's christening and she made it a very special day for Pauline and me. She was especially fond of my brother and really had a soft spot for him. I thought the world of her. Unfortunately we have lost touch with her since she later joined the Church and became a nun.

About nine months after the Rome salon opened, just when business seemed to be going really well, Bruno delivered a bombshell: he said he was unhappy working in Rome. He complained there were too many petty rules and it was very difficult to get the different types of licences that were needed. You had to know the right people and have the right contacts with different officials to be able to run the business smoothly. He had become upset and bothered by the complex bureaucracy and the low-level corruption. And he was frustrated that he was unable to deal with all this himself but had to leave it to Maurizio, who was born in Rome and knew all the officials.

Bruno felt like a fish out of water. He hated the sensation that he was not properly in control of his company. Although he was born in Italy, because Bruno came to England when he was so young, I believe that deep down he was very English in many of his attitudes. Italy might have been his home country but he did not feel remotely at home there. 'Toni, I don't feel as much

Italian as I thought I did,' he told me. He liked the simple and easy ways that he was used to in England. Business in Italy was much less direct. He didn't feel that Italy was to be his future or that it would fulfil the dream he had hoped for. He decided to return to London.

I think when you arrive in a new country sometimes you adopt the national philosophy and become more extreme than the people who were born there. Bruno liked things to be absolutely correct. He was very precise and well-ordered and very English in his own way. And above all, he was very ambitious. Even then his main aim in life was to be very, very rich. He wanted to be head of his own company and in charge of his own destiny.

Maurizio was devastated by the news. For him it was a great deal more than the breakdown of just another business relationship, he absolutely adored Bruno. He was in awe of him and, whatever happened, Bruno couldn't do anything wrong in his eyes. More than just a friend and colleague, Bruno was his idol and in a moment Maurizio's whole world came tumbling down. He was broken-hearted and Bruno's decision to walk out almost gave him a nervous breakdown. Maurizio's wife Teresa was quite a strong girl and very proactive; she moved in and took over on his behalf. She took charge of the situation and as I struggled to cope with the fallout from my brother's departure from Italy, all of a sudden I found that I had become 'public enemy number one'.

Everything was my fault in Teresa's eyes. Somehow she considered it was nothing to do with Bruno. I don't really know why, perhaps it was because they couldn't blame Bruno, so they blamed me. I would not have minded pulling out of Rome if they had done it properly, but Bruno would not wait. Once he had made his big decision he straight came back to England and started working in Sloane Square. He worked with David Mercer, who was an art director of the salon. David was hoping to open our first franchise in Brighton at the time but it did not materialise at the time. David later moved to Singapore, where he has built up a tremendous business for Toni & Guy.

The Sloane Square salon was busy and profitable and it worked very well for Bruno. A talented hairdresser, he worked extremely hard to build the salon but I think deep down, he was ready to start a new life in America. A few months later his dream came true and he was awarded a contract from KMS to promote their new product line in the United States and Bruno with the Toni & Guy Artistic Team was awarded a fantastic contract to carry out forty-eight shows throughout the United States.

The owner, and one of the founders, of KMS is a biochemist of Italian origin called Jamey Mazzotta, who resided in Redding, California. It was an amazing opportunity for Toni & Guy and for Bruno. But while he was in America grasping this great new opportunity, and living and achieving his dreams, the unhappy task of sorting out the end of the Rome salon was left to me.

It was a very difficult time. The Rome salon had been extremely profitable but pretty soon I had a message from Maurizio's wife Teresa to say that the profits were down. Suddenly there was only a small amount of profit and then, little by little the messages came through that there was no profit at all. Soon afterwards Teresa said the salon needed more money – she started 'squeezing the lemon', she was in control. The sole administrator of Toni & Guy, she was the only one who could sign for things. She took charge of everything and even tried to trademark the name Toni & Guy in Italy. It was very difficult to unravel the Rome problems and it became a horrendous situation. There we were with a stylish Toni

& Guy salon in the capital of Italy and it was completely out of our control. It was a nightmare. Teresa said she was losing more money and we would have to put more money in. I felt that Teresa and Maurizio had it in for me. After all, their relationship had been with my brother Bruno. They had no connection with me, no chemistry with me and that quickly became a big problem.

In the end my bitter and acrimonious battle with Maurizio and Teresa dragged on for eight years. During that time I had to attend courts and tribunals in Italy at least four times a year to try to sort out the salon and stop them using the Toni & Guy name. The late Vincenzo Lusa, who was a friend of our family and a very talented hairdresser himself and businessman, came to the rescue and attended all the meetings and tribunals with me he never knew how much help and support and confidence he gave me. He was a real rock.

Eventually at the end of countless meetings the tribunal ruled that Maurizio and Teresa could no longer use the Toni & Guy name, plus we agreed that to settle the matter they would pay us some money for our initial investment and in return they could keep the salon in Via Frattina. But before the agreement was finalised, Bruno arrived from America for a visit to Rome and decided they could have the salon back for nothing; he felt that he had achieved a great settlement. He was always very generous and supportive and I suppose quite forgiving. Of course later on Maurizio even visited Bruno in America and they continued their friendship, which is a great end to this particular story.

I suppose my eight years of battle did at least contribute to something special.

CHAPTER TEN

VENEZUELAN VENTURE

Travel never bothered me as I always felt I would go to the ends of the earth for a good deal. But when I ventured to a remote South American capital city, it turned out to be a trip too far. It was early 1979 and our business was going really well. We were getting offers left, right and centre, and it felt as though we were living in a fantasy world of endless excitement and opportunities, when we had an offer to go to Caracas in Venezuela to do a hairdressing show. We had never been to South America before and it felt like an exciting new adventure. It seemed an interesting place to go and on top of that we were offered $8,000 to make the trip. Money was certainly no problem at the time as evidently Caracas was flowing with oil. We did not quite know what to expect, but on arrival we were given a warm welcome.

Some of the people we first met seemed very flamboyant and wealthy, although we soon saw there were also signs of a great deal of poverty. It was a fascinating country and there were many Italian people there, which helped me to feel a little more at home. One clearly well-connected local guy called Enzo, who hired us for the Toni & Guy show and the seminars, came to meet us at the airport. Indeed, to our total surprise he arrived on the plane to welcome us in person! To me that seemed very odd because we hadn't been through customs or passport control. I pointed this out and he said: 'Oh, don't worry, I'll see you through the formalities. I have lots of friends and nothing is a problem when you know the right people in the right places.'

He did just that, ushering us off the aircraft and out of the airport as if we were important VIPs. I have to say we felt very, very important. It was almost as if we were world-famous superstars, and that's a great feeling. Enzo took us to see some elegant shops and on a small tour of Caracas. I soon saw that we had arrived in a very different kind of city from the ones we were used to. There was a lot of security at all the houses and shops, and when you visited a shop or hairdressing salon you had to ring the bell before you were carefully admitted. One guy's place we visited had a kind of fortress surrounding the property. Again, even more than when I had first arrived in Dallas, I felt I was in the Wild West – very exciting in one way, but also extremely scary. There were hugely wealthy people living close to desperately poor families, who we could see existed in total squalor. It was a city of enormous contrasts.

Our hosts were generous and friendly, and when we put on our first hairdressing show it went very well and I was delighted. I don't think the Venezuelans had seen anything quite like it before. We did a performance and afterwards we sold a lot of products, including all of the scissors we had brought with us. It was very encouraging, and I thought, *This is great, maybe there is a real opportunity for future business here.*

As our visit was nearing its end, Enzo approached me and asked if I could supply him with another fifty pairs of Japanese scissors. I quickly estimated that they would cost me about $3,000, but with that outlay I could make a return of at least £6,000 and double the money with one deal. Enzo said he didn't want to give me a letter of credit because it was 'difficult and complicated and the bank was not supportive'. I said that I needed to be paid up front. 'OK, why don't we do cash on delivery?' he suggested. At the time Pan Am flew into Caracas and they said that they could handle the delivery. It was something they did every day with no problem. As always, I was concerned about getting my money, but Pan Am assured me it would be OK. They said: 'If we don't collect the cash, we don't release the goods.' So I agreed to the deal and told Enzo we would be sending the scissors as soon as possible. I felt very secure that everything would be straightforward without any problems of any kind.

I bought the scissors in Japan and had them sent them to Caracas. I was told they had arrived at customs in Venezuela. A week or so went by, then another week, and although I waited patiently, nothing happened. So I phoned Enzo. He explained that he was desperate to receive the goods. I pointed out to him that my information was that they had been waiting at customs for nearly two weeks. What was the problem? He was very apologetic and said he'd go and collect them immediately from the airport. That obviously convinced me that everything was still perfectly fine. Then mysteriously more and more time went by and I received more and more messages that the scissors had not been collected. So I phoned Enzo again and he said the same things all over again. He was full of apologies and had more and more excuses for the delay.

It was all very strange. More time went by and Pan Am wrote to me and told me that the scissors had still not been collected. They could not understand what was going on any more than I could and asked what I wanted them to do. Should they bring the scissors back? I thought, *Well, in all honesty, what else can we do?* But the man from Pan Am said: 'There is a little problem. They've been here nearly a month and because they have gone through customs the customs officers will charge 100 dollars a day for storage!' That was then some 3,000 dollars, plus the cost of bringing them back. Of course my expected profit had disappeared on top of the initial investment. In order not to lose any more money I decided to abandon the scissors and leave them in customs in Caracas.

I realised that I had been duped: dishonest and slimy, Enzo was also a very clever operator. I felt such a fool to have been tricked by such a dishonest and dishonourable person – his behaviour was absolutely disgraceful. He might have made a little bit of cash but at the end of the day he lost me as a friend. I guessed he'd got the scissors and I let him know that I was very upset. I also told him that he could have made ten times more money if he had done business with me the honest way. It was a real shame and he lost an opportunity for both of us as well as ruining the chance for Toni & Guy to generate future business and profits in a new country. Well, it was a huge lesson for me to have learnt and unfortunately it has been repeated again and again in different circumstances in my business life.

I later realised exactly how he was working and how he got the scissors. I remembered when he came on the plane and how he knew everyone – customs officers, police and the airport staff. It would have been very easy for him to collect the scissors once they had been left, by explaining to the customs officers that he knew personally that the scissors would probably not have had much value, maybe a maximum of 50 dollars. It would have been an easy decision for the officer to dispose of them for some cash.

I have never seen Enzo since.

CHAPTER ELEVEN

FIRST FRANCHISES

The idea of franchising had been nestling in the back of my mind for a long time. Visits in the 1980s to Japan and later to Hong Kong, Singapore and particularly to the United States had shown me that it might be the way our business could best develop and grow.

But in England at that time no one really knew anything about franchising. Indeed when I went to to see my bank manager to ask him for some advice and to hear his thoughts on franchising, I was in for a big surprise. I thought franchising would be a great opportunity for my business and for Toni & Guy. Well, this particular visit to the bank was an experience I will never forget. My bank manager didn't really want to talk very much about franchising at all and did not seem to have an opinion on it; he was much more interested in asking me if I had a business plan or if I wanted a loan. He was also aware that my business was doing very well at that time and Toni & Guy was becoming increasingly profitable. I was excited but I wanted advice and backing and support for my new idea. Unfortunately, he had other ideas. He was a typically old-fashioned bank manager of the sort widespread at the time. Instead of warmth and wise counsel he was very unhelpful and cold towards me. I remember he had little glasses and he peered at me over the top of them in an intimidating manner. It was a very chastening meeting for a young hairdresser.

Nevertheless I stuck to my guns and told him my idea about growing my business through franchising. Carefully I explained that I had just come back from America and had seen that franchising was becoming huge in the United States and I told him that we should act quickly on this before I got left behind. And would you believe that after I had explained it all to him and spelt out my enthusiasm for my great idea to develop more Toni & Guy salons, he still wasn't at all interested. At the end of a highly unsatisfactory encounter he just offered me a loan and more or less told me that I was wasting his precious time! Unimpressed, I was determined not to let one man's ignorant opinion put me off my idea.

It is amazing what benefits come with travelling and how much people and things that you see in different parts of the world can broaden your horizons and provide so many new ideas and opportunities that even the professionals that we look up to, like our bank managers, get left behind. I was gradually learning that the so-called experts were often not nearly as expert as they thought. And more important, I was slowly building up the confidence to back my own judgement against that of others, even when the advice was very, very expensive.

A few months later, when this unhappy episode with my bank was still rankling, I was working in Davies Street on one of my busiest days. At that time I would do twenty to twenty-five clients a day and often I did not have the chance to have too much of a conversation. But just by pure coincidence while I was cutting the hair of one of my regular clients, a handsome young man in his mid-thirties came into my salon. He looked very trendy and we started chatting. I quickly warmed to this outgoing newcomer, especially when he told me that he was the new manager of Barclays Bank in Mount Street. I was a little unsure of him at first because he seemed completely different from the much older previous bank manager who had rejected my franchising thoughts so quickly. The man from Barclays was much more open-minded and after we talked for a while he said that if I was interested in a proposition, he had a very good deal for me.

At first of course I laughed at him because not for one minute did I believe him. I could not imagine he was genuine. I mean, after all, he looked nothing like a bank manager in any way, shape or form! He was far too normal and very natural, not stiff and difficult to engage with like the bank managers I had so far had the pleasure of encountering. So I said to him: 'Are you having a laugh with me? I know what a bank manager looks like and you certainly don't look like a bank manager to me!' He smiled and pulled out his business card. Lo and behold, he was indeed telling the truth – he really was the new manager of Barclays Bank on Mount Street. 'Oh, my God!' I said: 'You are a real bank manager.' 'Yes, Toni, I am,' he replied. Now that we had cleared things up he then proposed that I join his bank and if I did, he would give me free banking for two years with no charges. I thought to myself, *That's a bloody good deal*; it was an offer I couldn't refuse.

Everything seemed to happen very quickly in those days. We were getting offers and opportunities from every angle. It was an extremely exciting time for us. Of course I accepted the offer and being the opportunist that I am, I thought, *What have I got to lose? I get two years free banking and after the two years I'll go back to my old bank and ask for the same deal!* Unfortunately real life is not like that. In a fantasy world maybe that would have happened but I am still with Barclays today.

Determination and consistency have always been my strong points. I believe they are two of the most important qualities for any entrepreneur to possess. And I knew if we got it right then franchising could be one of the ways forward for our business. At that time no one knew anything about franchising in Great Britain. Wimpy Bars were spreading, and I think there were one or two McDonald's but the idea of franchising as a successful business technique was then still almost completely unknown.

Our first move into the world of franchising came in the early 1980s with a hairdresser who passionately wanted to open a Toni & Guy salon in Leicester, where he lived. He had worked with us for a while in Toni & Guy on Davies Street and wanted to take back to his hometown what he was learning in London and. So, after a few months' preparation, we opened the new salon in Leicester. Unfortunately it was not a success. I think it was perhaps a bit premature and we had no real structure in place. It was more of a good idea not fully thought out and sadly it quickly fizzled out. However, I had by then learned the fine English maxim, 'If at first you don't succeed, then try, try and try again', so instead of dampening my enthusiasm this experience just made me more than ever determined to prepare properly and open another franchise. Another reason for my determination to get it right was primarily that in those days I used to have a large number of stylists working for me. In Davies Street alone I had twenty-four, and almost all of them had got to a level where they could not further their careers or earn any more money: they had gone as far as they could go.

I was faced with a situation in which I knew most of them would emigrate, change careers or just give up hairdressing so we would have to replace them with new young, eager hairdressers. To me this seemed such a waste. I thought there must be a better way and that's when I became convinced that franchising would be the ideal solution because they could still carry on with Toni & Guy but own their own business. It would be profitable for everyone involved because we could share our images, uniforms, advertising and all of the tools of the trade. So that's how franchising became so firmly implanted in my brain.

Of course England was still quite different from the United States, where franchising was widely established and largely very successful, but I took the idea and adapted it to suit my business. There is always a reason and a need to do things. At that particular time we needed franchising for Toni & Guy because it was the only way I could keep my most loyal and valuable members of my team. This was not a revolutionary idea that I inspirationally came up with one night, but much more of a practical solution that filled a double need for my business. It retained the valuable talent that we had trained, and it developed Toni & Guy on the high street.

In spite of the Leicester experience I still had faith in franchising, but like life, business does not always turn out exactly as we might anticipate. There was at that particular time an excellent hairdresser called Peter Anthony Utolosky, who was the assistant manager of our Davies Street salon. Peter was a very hard-working employee, who always seemed to be full of energy and enthusiasm and had become a really good stylist. He desperately wanted to progress and create a career for himself and the idea of opening a Toni & Guy franchise salon became an exciting proposition for him. I thought he would be the best person to take on the challenge so together we opened the first proper Toni & Guy franchise salon in Twickenham in 1984. We made an agreement that he would run the franchise for an initial five years.

It seemed like a good move from the start as initially it all went really well, but business is often never as simple as you would like. I would later learn to my cost that I hadn't got the right handle on the franchise letting of the salon premises, because in those days landlords were not yet aware of franchise under-letting. Peter took on the lease under the name of Toni & Guy Twickenham owned by Peter Utolosky, but the landlord required my guarantee so I duly guaranteed the lease. The new salon became very successful straight away; it was the first proper Toni & Guy franchised salon in the UK. Peter was a good hairdresser and he had hairdressers coming from all over England, who wanted to work for Toni & Guy. At that time there were only three Toni & Guy salons and with Twickenham being the first franchise there was a lot of interest.

It worked very well for us and for Peter and the salon was very profitable from the start – so much so that Peter indicated that he wanted to expand to a second salon in Kingston. But six months before the end of the five years he dropped a bombshell and said that he did not want to carry on with the franchise. It became clear to me that he thought he could go it alone and would change his name to Anthony (his middle name) and carry on the business as his own. He knew that people would think he was my brother Anthony of Toni & Guy, which would be a big a draw for him as my brother Anthony was building a great reputation as a top hairdresser. Peter was paying us a 10 per cent royalty and he was making a great deal of money. He had the advantage of all the benefits of the Toni & Guy image – the photographs, education and the great growing reputation of our brand – but he felt he could do his own training and photographs as well as his own advertising and make even more money for himself.

Of course we tried to stop him and talk him out of this move but there was nothing we could do as he had already made up his mind. He took the Toni & Guy sign down and changed it to 'Anthony Utolosky'. Already he had negotiated the second salon we were going to do together in Kingston and after he gave in his notice he continued to proceed under his own name. However, what Peter greatly underestimated was that from now on he had to prepare his own collections, hire his own models, and do his own advertising and his own education. We had fifteen years of hard-earned experience behind us in these areas and we worked to a very high standard. Of course Peter had none of that experience.

One example of his inexperience was that he decided to place an advertisement in *Vogue* magazine, one of the most expensive magazines to advertise in. It must have cost him a minimum of £40,000, which would have been double what his royalty cost to us would have been.

I could see that he was heading for an abyss, for total disaster. He was no longer Toni & Guy and suddenly many hairdressers did not want to work for him. Most of the hairdressers who had been originally employed wanted to work for Toni & Guy, not him. Our brand was really growing in popularity at the time and he not only lost staff but the majority of the clients too. I'm afraid it was a complete catastrophe for Peter, or Anthony as he came to prefer, but it was of his own making.

Very quickly he then ran out of money. He couldn't pay

the rent or the wages; he couldn't cope with anything and the business was fast running out of his control. Almost suicidal, he had already started his second salon in Kingston and he was left with no choice but to shut the salon in Twickenham and move to Kingston. However, we'd made a decision as a company also to open a salon in Kingston. Having lost the Twickenham salon, with most of its staff and clients, I felt that I wanted to give them an opportunity elsewhere and what better place than Kingston? Of course, a brand-new Toni & Guy salon being in Kingston did nothing to help Peter's salon and very soon after he lost this one as well. I believe ultimately he had no choice but to go bankrupt. He still kept the salon open and he carried on the business in the name of his wife but not for long and shortly afterwards the salon changed hands again.

In a way I was happy that it hadn't worked out for Peter because after all I had done for him I felt it was wrong that he thought he could do better than us and tried to become our competition. But then I thought to myself: *Well, it's his decision and he is paying the price for his actions.*

Sometime much later I happened to bump into Peter when I was in Chiswick. 'Hi, Peter, how is it going?' I asked. 'Fantastic!' he said, 'I have now given up hairdressing – I teach posture. It is amazing, it is brilliant!' *How funny,* I thought to myself, but I did not show this reaction of course and instead I warmly congratulated him on his new-found career.

Then to my astonishment I received a letter from the landlord asking me to pay the rent in Twickenham as I was the guarantor! I couldn't believe it, I had forgotten all about that and was instantly sent into a state of shock. Also, there was a company called Hair Associates who had got wind of this difficulty and they announced that they would be happy to rent the shop and relieve me from that responsibility. They were at the time always ready to take advantage of any situation. I was briefly tempted and I was very close to making a deal with Hair Associates when I thought to myself, *Sod it! You know what? I will run it myself!* So I asked the landlord if he would be happy to transfer the lease to my name so I could carry on the business and to my delight he reassigned the lease to my company and said that he was happy that we had decided to stay. So we reopened the salon and built it up again. It was a great achievement and gave me great satisfaction. I regard it as one of the best things I ever did and the salon is still there today.

The first franchise that I regard as a true Toni & Guy franchise was opened in Brighton by Darren Brewer in 1989. Darren is a totally dedicated member of my team and has worked with me from a young age. He was a fine example to others and really proved himself by opening, running and maintaining a fantastic business. Darren runs his salon exactly how it should be run, to perfection with passion, determination and total organisation and as a replica of what I have already created. A model franchisee, he was always one of the leaders in my team and he became the one that everyone else wanted to imitate. Certainly he is a hard act to follow.

My second true franchise was opened in Guildford by Tim Avory in 1989. Tim's salon was an instant success. Even though he hadn't worked with Toni & Guy for a long time he quickly adapted to our philosophy. Another example of a model franchisee, today Tim is involved in over twenty salons and has helped to open more than any other franchisee. Both Darren and Tim gave me all the confidence and strength that I needed to open more salons and to continue to do so over and over again.

They showed me that it was possible, and for that I owe a lot to them. The late eighties and early nineties were quite a busy time for Toni & Guy as we also opened Kingston and Kensington as company-owned salons.

However, this was the time when the economy collapsed and of course rents were still very high. With Kingston I had a difficult rent review situation with the council who owned the property. The rent was about £16,000 a year but there was a review from two years earlier that unfortunately still had not been finalised. The estate agent informed me that in his expert opinion it would go up to a maximum of £22,000 or so. In the meantime the National Coal Board's pension trust had taken over from the council as landlord and they asked for an annual rent of £36,000! It came as a nasty shock to me. At that time I was advised by my estate agent that we had no choice but to go to arbitration and he was hopeful that in doing so we would be able to bring the rent down by a considerable amount.

So we went to arbitration and to my total amazement the arbitrators decided that two years earlier the market rent would have been £47,500! So even though the economy had totally collapsed and at that time the rent shouldn't have been any more than £22,000, you still had to pay the full £47,500. We were two years down the line so we had thousands of pounds of back rent as well as this huge new rent, plus the expenses and interest. All in all, I faced a bill of about £80,000.

I called the landlords from the Coal Board to have a meeting to see if we could make some type of deal. To my horror, I met a young man who was quite cocky and full of himself and did not appear interested in any deal whatsoever. He just kept saying: 'If the arbitrators had gone in your favour, would you have paid more?' Then he added: 'But nevertheless I will try to help you out and I'll give you this offer only once. I will let you pay us over a period of two to three years at 22 per cent interest and you can take it or leave it!'

I had no real choice – I had to take it because the future of the whole company was depending on it. This deal tied into our holding company, Mascolo Ltd. At one point I threatened to close the salon and walk away but then I learned to my horror that I could not do that without risking the whole business. We got through it all in the end, but it was quite an unnerving experience. Fortunately at that particular time America was doing much better than we were in the UK so I got a bit of help from them so I was really happy that our company had expanded in America; Guy and Bruno sent me some money as a matter of urgency. Many other groups and chains of hairdressing companies unfortunately were not so lucky, and some famous brands went bankrupt, so in a way I was very thankful and thought luck and God were on my side at that particular time.

It's been a continuous problem in our business: rents going up and increasing to a level in the boom years and then continuing at that high level at the time of recession. Always it creates a huge problem and in some cases if you haven't got enough funds it can make you bankrupt. These are the kind of lessons I am learning over and over again.

★　★　★

Fortunately in business as in life there are lots of silver linings behind the clouds of trouble. Perhaps one of the most wonderful things about being a hairdresser is that you find yourself meeting all sorts of interesting people. The famous movie-maker Ilya Salkind, who co-produced the *Superman* films with his father Alexander, was a client of mine for a long time. I feel very proud and lucky to be able to meet such amazing people and I was in particular awe of such a talented young man who was extremely down to earth despite all his success, fame and wealth.

One day when I was cutting his hair in Davies Street, Ilya told me about his ex-wife. He had been married to a lady from Los Angeles whom he had recently divorced. Ilya was telling me that he was worried about the fact that he no longer had much contact with his children and that his ex-wife was continually asking him for money. He seemed to be very stressed that his relationship had disintegrated to such an extent and he was extremely unhappy about the whole situation. The marriage hadn't gone well and the whole thing had gone wrong for him; I felt extremely upset and sad for him. I guess it's just one of those things that you hear when cutting someone's hair, as they do say a client tells his hairdresser everything, but this story in particular touched me more than others.

Ilya lived in nearby South Audley Street, although he also had houses in Los Angeles and Paris. A very gifted guy, he was always nice, friendly and a really open person, who usually seemed very easy-going and relaxed. I was happy that someone of his calibre treated me almost like a friend rather than just his hairdresser. Over the years I got to know Ilya really well as I used to do his hair often. With his marriage troubles, he decided to concentrate on his work and was making a lot of movies. He was always spending time with very famous actresses and he used to say they were extremely spoilt and always wanted their own way. For him it wasn't a real world, it was more like a fantasy world. He often told me that it was such a relief for him to come to the salon and be in the real world, to see all these normal, young, attractive girls. Ilya truly enjoyed the experience in Toni & Guy. I am sure he would really have liked to meet a 'normal girl' as he called them and although he was always telling me I was surrounded by lovely girls in the salon, he never actually made any advances towards them. He was a real gentleman.

This experience was such an eye-opener for me as I learned that it doesn't matter how rich or famous you are, we can all get a bit lonely and unhappy at times. One morning I was on my way to Davies Street for my usual appointments when the receptionist from the salon called me to tell me that there was a rather strange man sitting unshaven and half asleep in the middle of our reception area and she didn't know how to approach him. She thought that perhaps someone lost had wandered in and she was very concerned.

As soon as I saw him I recognised my millionaire friend and client, even though he did look extremely scruffy and unkempt. 'It's Ilya Salkind, he's a film producer!' I said. I rushed over and asked him how he was, offered him his usual cappuccino and invited him to the dressing-out position so I could cut his hair. He apologised for his appearance and he said he had had a very bad night and he was going through the worst nightmare he had ever experienced.

Superman films normally launched in the US and were fantastic box-office hits but when he produced *Supergirl* and launched it in London in 1984, the papers didn't give it the same promotion as he was used to receiving in the US, so he wasn't as successful. Not launching it in the States had been a huge mistake. He must have been really upset with himself and lost millions and millions of dollars overnight, so you can imagine how the poor guy might have felt. For me it seemed like for a moment I was part of history in the making, but there wasn't much I could do except give him some moral support and maybe offer him another cup of coffee!

I felt really sorry for him because he was such a lovely person. After this I didn't see him for a while and I wondered how he was and how his life was. You do get attached to your clients and you care for them. I was so excited when I saw he had made a booking in our Sloane Square salon. It was about six months since I had seen him and he brought in a delightful young lady with him and asked me to give her a completely new look: he wanted me to create something especially for her. Clearly he was very fond of her and I had a feeling he was going to marry her. He had remarried but had been divorced from his second wife for a year; this time, he explained to me, he was sure the lady was right for him. 'You must understand, Toni,' he said to me. 'Sometimes you go out with girls and you wonder if they really love you or if they love you for your money. It always gives me that insecurity but this time I am sure that she wants to be with me because she loves me, not my money and she probably has much more money than I have. She is one of the daughters of Charlie Chaplin!'

He looked very, very happy and satisfied with himself. I gave the young lady a brand-new haircut and did my upmost to do the best work that I could as I was very excited to cut the hair of such a famous woman and I was also so grateful to Ilya that he had introduced me and entrusted me to do his new girlfriend's hair. I had tremendous respect for him as a producer and also as a person. After he got married they moved to Paris, where she lived. Sadly, I've never seen him again since then but I often wonder how he is doing.

CHAPTER TWELVE

TRADEMARK TRIBULATIONS: TIGI IS BORN

One of the many lessons I have learned in business is that when everything seems to be going wonderfully well there is often an unpleasant surprise waiting for you just around the corner. Fortunately, hope often springs quite swiftly out of despair. Experience has taught me that normally after a disaster another opportunity presents itself quite soon. In spite of that optimistic outlook I found it was very hard to see the silver lining in the cloud that descended over us the day in the early 1980s when we received a devastating letter from the legal department of the extremely powerful and internationally successful Gillette Company.

It arrived just a couple of weeks after a memorable day at Salon International when we had launched Toni & Guy Gel. I will never forget how very excited I became, thanks to the warm initial reception to our exciting new venture. I saw some tremendous opportunities opening up for us in the future. Our product was astonishingly well received by all the hairdressers and I was thrilled that we were making an instant impact on all our latest styles: plaiting, weaving and hairstyles in gel shapes. I could see that there was enormous potential for some significant sales success in countless new markets all over the world.

The Gillette letter changed all that at a stroke. In no uncertain legal terms it spelled out that we had to withdraw all our Toni & Guy hair products because Gillette had trademarked the name 'Toni' in Class 3 (Cosmetics and cleaning preparations) so we should therefore not be selling Toni & Guy products, not even in our own salons! (Over thirty years before, in 1948, Gillette had acquired the Toni Home Perm company.) All my hopes came crashing down. I just could not believe what the letter was plainly telling me and I could not understand why we had no choice just because they had the trademark of Toni. We had been using Toni & Guy since 1963. It seemed ludicrous and totally unfair when we had proudly had signs stating Toni & Guy over the salons ever since we started the business.

Of course I took legal advice myself, but not for the first time it was all bad news. In our meeting with an expensive lawyer we were told very plainly that we had no choice but to agree to stop using the name Toni & Guy unless we wanted to go to court and challenge Gillette. I was told that this would cost us a minimum of half a million pounds and we would almost certainly lose the case anyway. Of course I did not have that sort of money at that time. If I'd had half a million pounds as a hairdresser then I think I would probably have retired straight away and gone back to live in Italy for the rest of my life. I was still young and inexperienced and I felt I could not take on a huge company like Gillette in a legal battle.

I took my counsel's advice after he gave a different example of a case in Switzerland where there had been a John Williams and a John Robert Michael and it was the first name that counted as being more important in the trademark and that vetoed the case of the second John. After that first name you could apparently have as many words as you wanted. It didn't make any difference. I said that our two names were together in Toni & Guy, which surely made it completely different but my counsel said that in his opinion it would be an almost impossible case for us to win in court. I was advised to remove the name Toni & Guy; I couldn't even use it for products in my own salon. Using my own name was illegal! That's what the lawyer told me, so that was the end of that.

So because of my relative inexperience and the unfortunate absence of half a million pounds in my bank account I had to accept his recommendation. Later I discovered this was not at all the right advice, which I came to learn was not remotely unusual from lawyers! Since then I have learned not to believe what lawyers tell you and to rely on your own judgement. My rule is to do the opposite to what the lawyers say and, usually, I come up trumps – I am not joking.

This was a shattering blow that seemed deeply unfair, but I believe it is important to recover from setbacks of all kinds as quickly as possible. At this time I felt very raw and cheated, but determined not to be beaten. Very soon afterwards we were at a show and I had a meeting with my accountant, Mr David Burke, and Dax Uinagi, the representative of Takigawa, the Japanese company I spoke of earlier, when I came up with an idea to overcome Gillette: we would change the name of our products. I was keen to retain as much of our identity as possible so I suggested we change the name to TIGI, using the Italian pronunciation of the initials of the names of my brother Guy and myself. I first went for 'TG' and because of the Italian pronunciation, I added an 'I' to each initial, spelling it TIGI.

And so TIGI was born as a product line registered in Trademark Class 3. It was the closest to Toni & Guy we could possibly get. I was happy that it identified very much with Toni & Guy, so that is what we created. We had to check with the lawyers yet again, much to my irritation, but eventually it was decided TIGI was acceptable where Toni & Guy was not. The funny thing is that a bit later, I was just thinking to myself, *OK, so we got that, and at least we are guaranteed that no one else can use Toni & Guy in the world.* No one, I believed, could ever come up with Toni & Guy products because Gillette would always police their trademark name. How wrong can you be? Because, I discovered, in Italy, Maurizio's wife Teresa had trademarked Toni & Guy as Class 3 for products. So I phoned Gillette and said: 'Surely you can get rid of this, like you did with me?' The answer came: 'I don't think we can do anything about it. It would have to be you who should police the name yourself!' I was astonished.

To be honest, they admitted, in Italy, Toni and Toni & Guy had never been accepted as the same thing. You can imagine the shock that ran through me. It seemed the law was available only to people with the largest chequebooks! I learned to my cost that you should never expect the law to be fair: expect it to be complicated, long-winded and extremely expensive, certainly but don't rely on fairness, because in my experience you will almost always be sadly disappointed if you do.

Years later there was a happier footnote to my legal defeat at the hands of the great Gillette. Over time their Toni perm became much less successful and they stopped using it, so then we attacked to get our name back. Things had changed enormously by this time. We had enjoyed considerable success, which was reflected in our bank balance, and I would have been happy to spend not just half a million pounds, but perhaps even two million pounds, to get my name back. I never thought I would ever get the name back but I never stopped wanting it. I kept trying and wondering how we could do it. Eventually we realised that they weren't using Toni any more and someone said: 'You might have a chance via "non-use".'

Naturally they reacted very negatively to our first approach and it looked as if it meant us going to court and fighting an expensive legal battle all over again. But that did not stop me for by this time I was very determined. They spent a lot of money building up their case but in the end they miraculously saw sense and decided they didn't use Toni any more so they were happy to let it go! I was pleased – I like happy endings.

★　★　★

I realised the importance and the tremendous potential of products and that became my focal point. It became very important to concentrate and make the best products with the right ingredients and create the type of line that would complement and help our style. I also realised we must do everything we could to make our packaging look young, fresh and trendy. As I've mentioned before, Toni & Guy was buying and selling lots of Japanese scissors. At that time I decided that we should have Japanese scissors, which would be different and exclusive to us so I designed a new style of professional scissor with a short handle, which gave much more control to the hairdresser. I then placed an order to Dax Uinagi for Takigawa to manufacture on our behalf our first TIGI scissors,

MK1 and MK3, 5 and 6 inches, made in Japan from a particularly hard kind of steel that would keep the blades sharp as a razor for years. Today, most hairdressing scissors in the world bear my design.

It was the time of twisted plaits, weaving and samurai shapes. We took advantage of these trends that we had created to introduce extreme and strong products like hair gel, highlighting gel and colour gel that worked instantly. We also introduced TIGI rollers, sort of bending rollers that provided an easy way for clients to create waves in their hair at home. They were available through mail order and advertised in free magazines like *Girl About Town* and *Ms London* and it was a great success.

I remember spending hours with my first secretary, Maria Carabine, opening thousands upon thousands of letters, with cheques and sometimes money stuffed inside them, at St Christopher's Place, our first academy, and then staying very late to pack thousands of TIGI rollers in Jiffy bags the same evening. It was an amazing experience and very satisfying and motivating. I have never minded hard work and Maria was a very loyal worker; she also worked hard for long hours. She was my assistant at first and quite a spirited girl. I remember she was so annoyed after I once chose another girl to do some blow-drying that she said: 'I'm going to take a course as a secretary and when I've passed all the tests I can be your secretary.' She never felt that she would be good enough to be my assistant and even with all of my persuasion and assurance that she would make a great hairdresser I could not change her mind.

Everyone had been saying that I should spend more time in the office being a businessman, so I made the decision to spend every Thursday there, even though it was my busiest day and I would take an average of £700 a day. First, I tried to do it all by myself and spent some time in the office in Davies Street. But it would take me all day to do two or three letters and they were awful. So I came to the conclusion that I could hire a secretary and at that time the average wage was £100 a week and cover her whole month's wages with just part of what I took on a Thursday in Davies Street.

First, I had a girl called Hazel, who was very clever and had been to university to study catering. She was brilliant, but she had studied catering and eventually decided to leave and open a restaurant. Then I decided to give Maria a chance for she was very driven and dedicated. We would stay behind until midnight or afterwards filling the bags with orders. People sent in cheques or cash and the money seemed to be flowing in from everywhere. It wasn't really enormous sums but it was very exciting.

Maria was a great employee and a great help to me, but then she left because my brothers started telling her what to do and she liked to take her orders from me and not from anyone else. As I said, she was spirited. She worked for a time with a firm of solicitors but then realised that she missed the atmosphere and the buzz of the hairdressing trade – and the excitement of going to all the shows. So after a couple of years she came to see me and asked if I would mind if she went to work for Trevor Sorbie even though she had left Toni & Guy years ago. I quickly agreed that she must be happy in her job and encouraged her to take up his offer and so she then went on and helped him to get his products into Boots. Eventually she came back to me and helped me to establish TIGI products and then finally started her own salon in Uxbridge.

★　★　★

We continued to perform in London and all over the world, doing hundreds of hair shows introducing our latest hairstyles, and I remember there was so much demand. One year, while my brothers were putting on a show at the Empire in Leicester Square and the rest of our teams were doing shows in other parts of the world, it was left to Pat, my hairdressing assistant at the time, and me to fly to Singapore for the first Toni & Guy show in that part of the world.

Our flight to Singapore was a terrifying experience. It was a really bumpy ride and we kept suddenly dropping hundreds of feet. I was petrified while Pat seemed to be enjoying herself as if she was at the funfair! *After this I can do anything*, I thought. As it happened, it was a very good Toni & Guy show. The event was a tremendous success. Our work was very innovative and extremely showy for the time but everybody seemed to love it. Pat was very talented at plaiting and weaving so we made a great double act. Afterwards we were practically besieged since everyone in the audience appeared to want to talk to us about our techniques and styles of cutting, as well as the academy in London. It was a fantastic experience that left me with a wonderfully warm feeling of great satisfaction.

I returned to Singapore nearly twelve years later for another show with a full Toni & Guy team, which was extremely professional, powerful and artistic. We put on a very strong and trendy show, but to my total surprise almost everyone I encountered was still talking about how fantastic the first show had been. They kept recalling the first time they met me with such excitement and enthusiasm that I was very moved. They all said they would never forget our first show.

We were travelling every part of the world and the next show was in Auckland, New Zealand. I travelled all the way from London for a one-day show and a one-day seminar with the Toni & Guy team. It was a totally different experience from what happened in Singapore. To me New Zealand seemed to be a beautiful country with strong British roots and lovely, attractive and very fit young people. Everybody appeared to be jogging through the streets of Auckland like athletes. I was very taken by their easy-going, outdoor way of life.

We put on an amazing Toni & Guy show right in the main hall in the centre of Auckland. We had hairdressers from all over New Zealand and even my very good friend, Luigi Giuliano, and his wife Judy came to see our latest collections and trends from London. It was a fantastic and truly memorable show. The next day we visited a few salons and then we did two teaching seminars that were fully booked. Everyone I met was amazed that I was not staying for another week to have a holiday and visit the country. After all, they kept pointing out, we had come from the other side of the world and it would have been a real opportunity but I was on a business mission, not a holiday, so I came straight back to London.

★   ★   ★

Probably one of the most important moments of my life was meeting Mr Kurt Andersen in London. He was a real gentleman from Copenhagen who became a trusted colleague and a true friend. An experienced and professional manufacturer, he owned a factory in Denmark that made hair products under licence from a Paris company called Eugène Perma, and had a great deal of knowledge about manufacturing business. He was extremely helpful and supportive and we hit it off straight away.

Kurt was almost a mentor to me, as Mr Feak had been earlier. He was extremely wise and kind. We both knew we could help each other and we quickly put together our first strong gel, peppermint mousse, shampoo and conditioner and highlighting gel (silver, gold and red), colour gels and very strong hairsprays that would work immediately on stage. They were innovative products and were immediately loved by many hairdressers. This helped us create our collection for that year and it was the start of a great friendship between Kurt and me. I remember in the late seventies we had an order for 25,000 tubes from Australia – that was our biggest sale of Toni & Guy gel with Kurt. Later we opened our first Toni & Guy Academy in Copenhagen to show our products in Europe and to teach the latest Toni & Guy techniques. Unfortunately under Danish law we could only have a lease for five years. After that we could not renew it.

As the demand grew we opened our first warehouse and offices in Chelsea Wharf under the administration of Jackie Lark. I remember employing a close school friend of David Mercer, a former art director at the salon, called Simon Cooper, an ex-British Army stock controller to run our warehouse and stock, which he did with military style and precision. I also employed two young reps to start our first distribution for the United Kingdom. In the office there was my PA Maria and Caroline supporting Jackie so we had a small team to run our distribution of TIGI.

Exports orders continued to grow; I remember receiving an order for £10,000 worth of gel for Australia and one for thousands of posters, books and videos for the USA and especially a huge order for posters from Russell Zims, vice president of KMS. That was a fabulous order! And this happened after we toured all over the United States doing Toni & Guy shows on behalf of KMS, which created a huge demand for the posters and was the start of an adventure for our Toni & Guy accessories for the USA. So we concentrated on export orders for our TIGI products and Toni & Guy accessories as it was very profitable and I could see potential for a clear growth.

Realising that we needed a complete and full TIGI product line before we could run a team of reps for the UK, we decided to concentrate on selling our TIGI products and Toni & Guy accessories via mail order in the UK. Unfortunately our Chelsea Wharf warehouse posed a big problem: you couldn't park anywhere near it – well, not legally anyway – and we had constant battles with the traffic wardens that made life very difficult. We used to get parking tickets all the time when we were just trying to run a warehouse. How can you send orders out when you can't even park your van? It was ridiculous but despite all the difficulties it was the beginning of our real expansion.

It was time for Jackie Lark to return to St Christopher's Place to set up a new business venture. This was a 'video club' she ran with the help of Pat Sangster, who had had looked after the Toni & Guy account on behalf of Wella for nearly twenty years. The video club became another success for our business.

CHAPTER THIRTEEN

TONI & GUY
USA

Bruno worked in the Sloane Square salon for a while after leaving Rome and did some excellent work but he was always very ambitious and eager to get on in life so he never really settled. It was not long before he decided that his future lay in the United States of America. At this point I must go back in time and recap a little to explain our expedition to the world's richest country that was to change Toni & Guy forever. We left for Los Angeles in a small but enthusiastic party of four close friends and colleagues, who were all very excited to explore exciting opportunities in the States.

I will never forget the trip. There was Alan Doyle, who was our art director at Davies Street, Takigawa's agent Dax Uinagi, Bruno and myself. Determined that this trip would lead to something definite for us, I had already organised L1 work permits to allow Bruno and Alan to stay in the States for a certain length of time working for our company. With the help of our Japanese contacts we were hoping to open a Toni & Guy salon in California. Soon after we arrived in the sunshine we were introduced to a man who owned a salon on Rodeo Drive, probably the most luxurious shopping street in Los Angeles. In his late sixties, he had moved to the USA from Eastern Europe many years before and was very excited at the prospect of turning his salon into a Toni & Guy. But he had one rather surprising condition: before he slipped quietly off into retirement – he wanted to keep working for a while. And he wanted to do it with us, to be part of the Toni & Guy world! He suggested that he would like to remain and keep a chair in the salon for the next two years to look after his clients and enjoy and participate in the atmosphere of young and trendy hairdressers. Following this, he would then sell the salon to us for $2,000, which I thought was a real steal.

Alan was joyful at the prospect of the proposed deal but to my astonishment, Bruno wasn't nearly so excited. I thought Rodeo Drive would be just up his street, but he had some personal problems at the time and he didn't think it was the right time for him. So Alan stayed on in LA and later opened a different salon of his own and achieved his dream. Meanwhile Bruno returned to Oxshott, Surrey, where we lived, to sort his life out. But sometime later we had a visit from Paul Joseph, a very interesting young man who owned a salon in Hawaii, which I believe he told us he was on the verge of selling. He wanted to get more involved with Toni & Guy and was especially keen to work with my brother Bruno in the United States. Following on from that a friendship blossomed between us. Paul was quite a showman with a huge personality, and he went on to become a strong ally to Bruno in America.

A little later another opportunity came our way. KMS wanted to launch their product line and asked us to tour the USA doing Toni

& Guy hair shows in over forty destinations. Bruno took charge of the team and it was an enormous success. This marked a personal as well as professional high for Bruno, for he met a beautiful girl from Dallas called Terry, whom he married in 1982. They came to England, where they lived in Oxshott for a while. Guy and I were still living nearby and it was a wonderful time to be together again. We enjoyed living near each other very much and we used to meet regularly. They were very happy moments for me, especially as I had young children who were delighted to be close to their uncles and cousins.

Anyway, back to the US tour. Terry's mother was a real-estate agent in Dallas and business was booming. It was the time when America was covered with gold and she quickly gave Bruno the opportunity to buy a beautiful home worth hundreds of thousands of dollars, which the developer would sell to him without the need for a deposit. If you did not have the cash to put money down, you could have your constructed home without a jacuzzi. In that case they would deduct the cost of the missing jacuzzi and that could serve as your deposit! They would do almost anything to conclude a sale. For Bruno it was a great opportunity and a dream come true. I can't imagine that happening in England.

I always believed that the only way to establish and expand our business in the United States was to put down a strong foundation and open a Toni & Guy salon there. It was what we knew best and what we were confident at doing, plus we were very good at it. And Bruno was ready for it now: he decided it was the perfect moment for him and characteristically he wanted to go to America in style, so the company exchanged his car for a Rolls-Royce! We bought it in Switzerland, which we thought would at least mean the steering wheel was on the left-hand side so it would be fine for the USA. We still, however, had to pay an extra £1,000 for adjustments to make the car legal in America. The Rolls cost £12,000. Don't forget at that time the pound was close to parity with the dollar – the same car in the USA would have cost $50,000 or $60,000 dollars so it certainly raised a few eyebrows.

In fact, the Rolls-Royce proved a great success in helping the arrival of Bruno and ensuring that he and Toni & Guy made an impact. Americans seemed highly impressed and it proved to be very influential after Bruno was introduced to the local bank manager. We needed to get loans and Bruno had the crafty idea of asking his father-in-law to buy himself a cap and drive him in his beloved Rolls to the bank, so it seemed as if he was so wealthy and successful that he had already hired his own chauffeur!

At the meeting with the bank Bruno explained all about Toni & Guy and what a tremendous opportunity it was to expand in the United States with a brand already recognised in so many parts of the world and with family experience going back hundreds of years. He invited the bank manager for a meal and even had his father-in-law drive them to the restaurant in the Rolls! Of course after that performance the bank manager was deeply impressed and offered him half a million dollars as a loan with no guarantees. It was 1985, and the US economy was flourishing. With the help of Terry's close friends, an extremely wealthy South American family called Borja, along with other financial support and contacts, Bruno opened his first salon on Sherry Lane in Dallas. From start to finish his planning and strategy were excellent and within a matter of weeks he had built a busy salon. It was very profitable, very quickly. This first salon was quickly followed by two more in Dallas – one in Galleria and the third in Northpark Center.

This was the right time for Toni & Guy to bring to America

a new philosophy of hairdressing that was highly specialised in its use of a team of trained hairstylists, technicians and public relations people, all backed with a system of assistants. It was very different from the American way of working on commission, where hairdressers were also technicians and did their own shampoos, swept their own hair and on top of that, kept their own client records. This system had worked extremely well for many years but unfortunately it would not create any real artistic talent because hairdressers were doing a bit of everything and mastering nothing. Everybody told us that we would not be able to persuade America to switch from their system but we grabbed the bull by the horns and Toni & Guy changed hairdressing in America forever by maintaining the highest standards of education and creativity. It was a wonderful time.

Very quickly Bruno was at the centre of an incredible success. I often travelled to Dallas to give whatever help I felt was required and I was very proud of my brother's achievements, always regarding him as an extremely clever operator. I enjoyed every moment of my experience in Dallas and it was a great opportunity for me. It was at the time much easier to grow in the States than in the UK and so I decided for the benefit of Toni & Guy to capitalise the debt that was owed by Toni & Guy USA of £137,000 to the UK to give it that extra push.

So Bruno was doing very well in America and it was around 1986 when Guy decided that he wanted to cross the Atlantic to join him. Of course Bruno was happy to get more help from the brothers. Guy was very enthusiastic about the chance to start a new life and he realised, as I did, that America had huge opportunities for growth and he could accelerate his life so much quicker than if he stayed in the UK. Everything was just perfect for Guy; he knew it was the right moment. Just a short time later, my other brother, Andrea, took the same decision. Andrea was unable to be a hairdresser because of a slight paralysis in his right hand, but he had experience in the UK of working with BT and is very talented technically. He loved the opportunity to get involved in editing Toni & Guy films and videotapes and at the time it was crucially important.

An inspirational figure, Andrea greatly motivated others and helped to grow that side of the business. Like Guy, he has a fine personality and excellent interpersonal skills with the Toni & Guy staff. He and Guy were a tremendous support for the growth of the business and they were also a great help to Bruno in America. Very quickly, six or seven salons were opened in the States and the sales of TIGI products were growing rapidly in America.

After the successful tour with KMS that helped the company establish itself in the USA, Bruno started a conversation with the KMS president Mr Mazzotta about the possibility of them producing a product line for TIGI. We were invited to meet at their offices in Redding, California. I asked my trusted and very experienced friend Kurt Andersen, with his comprehensive knowledge of hair products, to come with us to give his advice. He promptly accepted, left Copenhagen and met me in London.

After joining Bruno, Guy and Anthony in Dallas we spent the day there and then left for Los Angeles, from where we boarded a small jet for Redding. On arrival at the offices of KMS we were warmly welcomed by our friend, KMS vice president Russell Zims, and after offering us a drink he became quite open. Previously he had spent a considerable amount of time with my brother Bruno on his Toni & Guy tour of America and they had become good friends. He warned us that we had a long wait, even though the board and the president were ready; evidently they used the waiting tactic to make guests feel awkward and nervous before any potentially difficult negotiations. Unimpressed, I responded by informing them politely that the meeting was not life or death to us and we could wait a lifetime and still not become agitated or unsure because we didn't need anything from them.

When they finally came to meet us they shocked me by saying they didn't want Mr Andersen to be included in our meeting. I thought this was extremely rude and outrageous. Furious, I wished to leave immediately and go back to London, but Mr Andersen being the gentleman that he was, even after having had by far the longest journey of any of us, insisted strongly that I joined the meeting. Although I argued with him, he wouldn't take no for an answer. And after a lot of persuasion I eventually agreed, but I was left full of bad feeling and I realised they were perhaps not the right people to do business with.

As it turned out our business relationship never did progress. In fact, it never really got started at all, but one good thing that came out of it was Mr Russell Zims later became Bruno's second-in-command: the vice president of TIGI USA. It was another important lesson that I learned about business on my long journey.

After a short spell based in Simi Valley in California we opened a warehouse in Dallas and by then I was spending more and more time in America. I was visiting three or four times a year, giving my support. At that time I still only had the two salons in London, in Davies Street and Sloane Square. I had to pay the tax on the money left in the USA as capital so therefore I found it was not possible for me to grow the business or open any more salons in London until after I had paid all of the tax. In the meantime I could see that our business in America was growing faster and faster, and it was a tremendous satisfaction for me to see such success.

It was not long before the directors of Toni & Guy USA realised that with the help of some of their investors they might as well take over the business in England. After all, they thought, as there were then only two salons and one franchise in the UK they could easily run them as one company from America. I am sure that at the time they must have felt this was in the best interest of Toni & Guy USA, however I must admit that it came as a real shock to me and it left me with a feeling of failure, also a sense of ingratitude for all the whole-hearted support and the real passion that I had happily given to Toni & Guy USA. Despite this I knew that their suggestions that they should take over the UK business had been made with the best of intentions. Nevertheless that was the fundamental moment in my life that inspired me to expand and grow the business in England, as well as in the USA – I have to thank Toni & Guy USA for that.

By that time Bruno's third wife Kyara had become involved in TIGI USA and I felt that she was very inspirational and extremely passionate about TIGI products and TIGI cosmetics. She had a real sense of creativity, especially for packaging. Later she became very much the power and the strength behind the rapid growth of TIGI USA and was a huge support to Bruno.

I made the decision to stop going to the USA so often as I didn't feel that my presence was required any more. My brothers did not need me as much as they once did, so I concentrated my energies much more in London and we opened our third salon in Covent Garden in 1988.

★ ★ ★

I clearly remember I started having doubts at the last minute. Is it really going to work? I wondered. Covent Garden was then an up-and-coming area, but for many years it had been the fruit and vegetable market of London, an exciting and interesting place, full of history (my father used to buy grapes that came from Puglia there to make wine in the fifties). Now it had become very fashionable, the 'in' place to be. We opened our salon and for the first three months it was unbearably quiet. I remember Brenda Mail, one of my most faithful and longest-serving employees, coming to give her support and also being worried about the prospects for the future. Brenda was remarkable – she treated Toni & Guy as her own company and never stopped to amaze me with her passion, professionalism and consistency as long as I have known her. She's been a rock, and was fundamental to the growth of Toni & Guy back then, continuing to play a vital role in the business even today.

Brenda and Jackie Lark have both been with Toni & Guy since the 1970s and are still as keen and enthusiastic about the business as ever. At a time when they might be considering retirement, both ladies seem to want to soldier on with me. I'm delighted but perhaps I should allow them to explain for themselves how they feel.

Jackie Lark says:

Toni has always been a wonderful man to work for, but at first I was quite fearful of him because I didn't know him very well. I was a single mother working from home, doing the books. It was not easy being on your own with children back then, but Toni was very kind and thoughtful. Even after I started working full-time in the office, once the children were at school, he would let me work from home during the school holidays. Not many employers were anything like so understanding in those days. And he was always very careful with his money. When I first worked with him in an office I can remember him walking round and proudly saying his shoes were thirty-two years old. And he wore the same blue winter coat for years. That became his trademark. He was very prudent.

I struggled as a single parent and my younger son Daniel was a bit lost. He had a very good education and I said to him, 'Why don't you think about hairdressing?' It's good to have a trade. I went to talk to Toni and though the company course cost a lot of money, he let Daniel do the course for nothing. That training gave Daniel a great step on the ladder and he is still in the business today, aged thirty-eight. Toni was very generous – I will always be grateful. He says Toni & Guy is like a family, and it is. He really believes it. He is so hands-on; he is involved in everything and he cares about everybody. He knows a lot about a lot of the people in his life. There are 250-odd salons in the UK, then all of the overseas salons, but he always seems to know what is going on.

Recently our franchisee in Japan, with whom we had worked for years, suddenly died. Toni was immediately over there, supporting the family. Even at his age he is very active. He got straight on the plane to Japan and supported them through the memorial service. He will always have his eyes and ears open. I always thought he would be successful because he worked so hard and had such high standards but I never dreamed there would be Toni & Guy salons all over the world. I think it's wonderful what he has created.

Brenda Mail says:

Toni is remarkable. Even at his age he works incredibly hard. In spite of all the success he is never one to travel first class. He is always happy in economy flights and he still gets the Tube and the bus or train to work. He wouldn't dream of getting a cab – he would be quite horrified at the waste of money. He works such long hours that I often try to make him have a driver to pick him up and take him home at the end of the day but he always says, 'No, no.' And just gets on the train and goes home.

He is not mean but he simply can't bear waste. In the early days when we passed a letter from one office to another in an envelope, we had to address the envelope in pencil so we could use it again! In the very first recession Toni conducted a real purge. Stationery, you could have but it couldn't be wasted. He would pick up paperclips or pencils from the floor and they would be used again. He hated to see waste, especially at a time when everyone was tightening their belts. That attitude goes in the salons as well: every haircut counts and every client has to buy a product. Toni made sure everyone knew resources were limited; he couldn't bear waste.

He has always been a very kind employer. He has always been strict but fair. But he is certainly not a pushover: if people are off sick and are genuinely ill, he is sympathetic but he has no tolerance of skiving. He is amazingly kind if anyone had a problem. I'm a good example of that myself – I've been ill for the last three years and he has been fantastic. He told me to take whatever time off I wanted and he and Pauline wanted me to come and stay at their home so they could look after me! As it happened I have been quite lucky and haven't needed to move in but I'll never forget their warmth and generosity.

He absolutely hates staff leaving. When anyone quits he

takes it very personally and gets very upset, and he always takes them back, whatever they've done. He is very forgiving, more than any of us.

He has changed people's perception of hairdressing. It is seen as a big business now whereas it wasn't before. It was lots of small businesses but when we went into franchising so successfully it became seen as a considerable business. And a lot of that is down to one man: Toni. I've never had an appraisal – I think we started one once, and his opening line was, 'Are you going to sit and tell me you're retiring?' And I said, 'No, have I got to retire?' He said, 'No' – and that was the end of it! There is a genuine family feeling to Toni & Guy. People try to make it corporate but it never works. Toni would be the first to break the rules. He's a great boss – I really respect him.

It is heart-warming to hear such remarks and I would also like to give a much younger employee, my hard-working PA, Michelle Dersookiasian, the opportunity to have her say:

I have learned so much from Toni – he is a kind and brilliant boss, who can be inspirational. He has taught me so much and I feel privileged to do a job I love. If there's an incident that sums Toni up, it is perhaps the time he went out to our Drayton offices and found a van parked in his space. Some bosses would have shouted the odds but Toni quietly parked somewhere else and later assured the van driver that his delivery was important so he did the right thing in parking in the boss's space. That's Toni!

CHAPTER FOURTEEN

NO TURNING BACK

Making a success of our Covent Garden salon was never easy. I depended a lot on Darren Brewer, who was the artistic director. He was a very creative and confident young man and we had a strong and dynamic Art Team. Everything was in place but at first it was just not happening. It was still very slow, and it was extremely worrying. And then suddenly, just a few weeks later, it all happened. Clients started to come back, and new and recommended customers followed. In a matter of weeks it became as busy as Davies Street and Sloane Square.

Toni & Guy had finally conquered Covent Garden! That was the turning point for Toni & Guy and franchising. Now there was no turning back, no stopping us and the growth of the business was amazing. We followed by opening the second franchise in Brighton with Darren in 1989, and Guildford in the same year and then in 1990 Bromley, Windsor and Richmond, followed quickly by Kensington and Kingston as company-owned salons in 1991. It was all go!

From the outside when everything is running smoothly it might look simple to run a Toni & Guy franchise. After all, it is a tried-and-tested formula and there is a proven demand. But I know very well that running one of our franchises is a difficult and demanding job. Fortunately it can also be enormously rewarding. I can't think of anyone better than my wife Pauline, who ran our Kingston-upon-Thames salon with great success, to explain exactly what it's like.

Pauline said:

It was really down to my poor mum that I took on the Kingston salon. Sadly, in the mid-1980s she was diagnosed with cancer and for the last eight months of her life she came to stay with us. My two oldest children had left school by then but Pierre, the youngest, was still at the Danes Hill School, which was right next door. Looking after my mum was a full-time job, bless her, but I am so pleased I was able to take care of her and make her last months as bearable as possible. It was not easy being a full-time carer and it certainly kept me busy.

And it was my mum who really made the decision for me to go back to work and take on a franchise. I had been considering going back to work as soon as Pierre went to Danes Hill. He just used to go through a gate in the garden fence and he was there, and he didn't finish a long day until 5.30 or 5.45 in the evening. I think Toni thought I should be getting back to work. He knew that I always liked to be busy and he thought that I would be bored if I stayed at home on my own all that time.

Everything changed after Mum developed cancer. It was awful, of course, but with hindsight I was so pleased I was able to look after her myself for those last eight months. We were very close and I had to be there for her. She was very brave throughout but we knew there was only going to be one end to it and we faced it together.

It was so very sad. All the time she was ill she knew that she was going to die. Then just before she died Toni was finally able to get the shop in Kingston. My mum said to me many, many times, 'When I go, I want you to go and take that shop on. It is for your own good and I know that you will make a great job of it.' After my mum died I did agonise about what to do and thought, *Shall I or shan't I?* Taking on a Toni & Guy franchise is a very big job, which comes with a huge responsibility and a great deal of effort and hard work, but in my heart I knew that my mum was right. She knew me very well and she knew that if I sat around the house moping on my own then I would just get upset. She knew I needed a job or something to do. Of course my mum was right: it was the best thing for me to do. I have always been the sort of person who is happiest when they're doing something constructive and useful, and starting up the Kingston salon was a real challenge.

It was my first time going properly back to work after having the children and, as any mother who is considering returning to work knows, you can lose a lot of confidence if you're out of the workplace for a while. I certainly found it hard to return to work. I felt very nervous and apprehensive and I did have some last-minute nerves and thought for a while that I wasn't going to go in that first morning because I thought I couldn't do it any more. After you have been looking after children and the home for a time, you begin to think that perhaps that is all you can do. It was a real wrench to get myself there that first morning.

But I just thought, *Well, I've got to go in now because the staff will all be waiting for me.* So I pulled myself together and went in, and within an hour or so everything flooded back to me. My confidence returned and I knew I had done the right thing. And forever afterwards if ever I occasionally faltered I could hear my mother's voice saying, 'When I go, do this for me.' That kept me going. To be honest, that first day was difficult, but afterwards it was fine.

I loved starting from scratch in a new salon. I would be in at nine o'clock every morning – there was always so much to do, but I love being with people and I love everything about good hairdressing salons so it was great. I tried to do everything as well as I could and one of the first things I concentrated on was building up the colour, or technical, side. Before long we had the best technical side in all our divisions, I literally made it the best. I was very proud of myself when that happened.

I wanted to make Kingston special. I'm not very good at making money, like Toni, but I do have a passion for doing people's hair and making them feel good – that I do share with Toni. I was always very hands-on. Even when I was in charge before I had felt I was just part of the team and I did all sorts of the lowest and dirtiest kinds of jobs. I was just the same in Kingston. Some of the employees in the salon were shocked when I insisted on doing everything, even down to a shampoo. I love hairdressing. If others were busy I'd do shampoo, cutting, blow-drying. That was because I knew how I wanted it and no one else did.

Clients are the most important people in the hairdressing world. If they go out happy, you've done your job. It's such a pleasure to see someone walk out happy, knowing you've made them feel wonderful. I'll never forget soon after I'd opened Kingston and I was trying to get everybody to share my feeling that customer is key. My message was always, 'When your client comes in, you've got to really love that person.' You see a lady coming in and you must think, I want her to look really special going out. You should visualise that as soon as they walk in, I believe. I used to hold a meeting every single morning to try to teach my staff exactly how they should be feeling about our clients: if they are feeling right, then it comes across in the salon. I would guarantee that if they followed my direction during the day then they'd be busy and I believe they all really liked to be busy.

We had only been open for about four weeks when we had a client who really made me feel we were doing something worthwhile. One day this grim-faced lady walked past the salon and instantly I thought to myself how sad and forlorn she looked. I saw her looking nervously in the window and then walk quickly away down the street. Then I saw her again, looking in, and then after a while she came hesitantly inside. I went over to reception because I wanted my receptionist to see how you should treat someone who is feeling perhaps a little nervous or troubled. I always wanted my staff to try to assess how our customers were feeling as soon as they came into the salon. I knew this lady was unhappy about something. She was very cautious and obviously not feeling very relaxed at all. I didn't want to rush her so I suggested she might like to come in for a consultation another day, and I gave her a card.

I said: 'See what you feel like and what sort of style you'd like. You don't have to pay anything for that.'

She took the card, left, and within ten minutes she was back in the salon again. She had clearly steeled herself to make a huge effort and she said: 'Can I have a consultation now?' I took her inside and got one of the girls to do it and I stood there watching. She asked if she could have her hair done, there and then. I said: 'Are you sure?' because she still seemed very nervous and fragile. She said she was sure now so we went ahead. We did an all-colour and cut and afterwards I was delighted to see that it looked great. If I could have taken before and after pictures of how she looked it would have shown the difference was incredible, but even better than the new hairstyle the smile on her face was the best thing we created. I was so pleased and I just thought how great she looked as she walked out of the shop.

The next morning this man came in with a box of chocolates and he said to me: 'I just want to tell you how much I appreciate what you've done for my wife.' He handed over the chocolates and proceeded to tell me she had just come out of hospital after treatment for a nervous breakdown. Her confidence had been rock bottom when she went out but she had come back with her new hairstyle feeling a great deal happier. He said: 'My wife came home like a different woman – she was so much more like her old self. I can't thank you enough.' I was delighted and I was so moved that I cried later when I got home. It's the sort of experience that makes your day.

You can go home and feel you've really made a difference to someone's life. It can be wonderfully rewarding, doing people's hair. Who's to say that in years to come you might not need someone to do that sort of thing for you? I always wanted people to walk out of the salon feeling *This is really great!* And that was what I always strived for in Kingston. Doing someone's hair is a very important, very personal and very fulfilling job. A good hairdresser can make a real change to the lives of some of their clients. People can relax and really be themselves and I love that contact the job brings. Toni and his brothers all knew that as they were brought up and I have learned it for myself.

But running your own salon can be very demanding. Once we had some young girls booked in who all wanted sixties beehive styles for a special party. The styles were from my era, though that night unfortunately I was having a dinner party at home so there was a potential problem as I would not be there to direct operations. But the girls in the salon were sure they could cope. They insisted I went ahead with my plans and said they could manage. I had to leave the salon at about four o'clock to get everything ready for the meal. I had just about finished preparing the food when the phone went. Beehives are not as easy as they might seem and the girls in the salon were really struggling. I did not think twice – I just put my coat on and went back to the salon for six o'clock.

Beehives were my speciality when I was younger and I put three girls' hair up while everyone was watching me. We managed to cope with all the clients and I was back home for my guests by quarter to eight. Everyone understood that things were running a bit late. I could just have said to the girls: 'Do it the best you can,' and left them to it, but I couldn't do that. Toni understood my decision perfectly – it is exactly what he would have done himself.

Hairdressing was always more than just a job for me. Occasionally I even did people's hair for nothing if I knew they couldn't afford it. Back in the Clapham days I remember one particular occasion when an elderly lady came in. I was cutting her hair and I could see that she really needed a perm so I suggested it to her. She said: 'I'm so sorry, dear, I haven't got the money.' I knew Toni would not approve of me letting her off paying but I couldn't see him anywhere so I gave her a perm and we just put it down in the book as a cut and set.

Afterwards Toni said to me: 'I thought she had a perm.' I said: 'Well, she did, but she couldn't afford it so I did it for nothing.' He said we weren't going to make any money if I did that very often – but for me it has never really been about the money: I love how you can brighten up people's lives. I had one lady who was in despair because a coloured style from another salon had gone horribly wrong. I improved it and she was happy, but I wasn't. I did it again so it looked fabulous and I didn't mind bearing the cost. To this day I've still got a few longstanding customers whose hair I do for nothing. I love it. Over the years they have become friends and it's nice I can afford to do their hair without charging.

Hairdressing is not like any other business. It is a very personal service that hairdressers provide. There is an element in our business where you feel like a psychologist as well because you want to please your client and be as kind as you can. There are only about three businesses in the world that you can actually get that personal with, where you can actually touch people. Doctors and nurses and other medical people have to be hands-on and so do masseurs, but hairdressers go to work when their customer is usually not ill or stressed but relaxed and receptive. You get very close to people and you can really help them sometimes. Then it can become very rewarding, and not because of the money.

I loved being a franchisee. Because all the brothers were together I didn't want to get involved in running the business as such, but the franchise was my sort of thing. I was in charge at Kingston and it was my little empire, so I did what I had to do. In fact, it went so well that Anthony, Guy and Toni said, how come she's made it so busy there, particularly on the technical, the colour side? That drew in a lot of extra money. I believed in it with a passion and I said we should have it throughout our company, which we did not have at that time. We are known for cutting but not for colour; we should be known for colour as well. Toni and the brothers agreed and so they asked me to start going to the school and start taking charge of colour.

I wasn't sure about going up to town. I had had Kingston for four or five years then when they asked me. Pierre was thirteen. He was leaving Danes Hill by then, and he hated his new school; he was so unhappy. He said he really wanted to go to acting school. I said: 'You're only thirteen.' But he knew his own mind and he said that acting was what he really wanted to do more than anything else in the world. I phoned the Italia Conti Academy of Theatre Arts in London. It was not easy for him to get in but he managed it and he had a brilliant time; he really shone. That freed me up to go to London every day and concentrate on the colour.

For several years I ran the colour division of Toni & Guy.

It was my passion. I really loved every minute of it, until gradually I set people up in divisions to take over from me; I wanted them to grow. Eventually I could slowly come out of that division. I finally gave up when Sacha had her baby, then I just wanted to be at home. Vito is eight years old now – family is always the most important thing for me.

CHAPTER FIFTEEN

TIGI WORLDWIDE

A s the business grew it became the right time for TIGI to take on more key staff. First, I employed a financial controller. I hired Terry Bellamy, a very together young man, who was an extremely competent chartered accountant, as well as being very self-confident. Soon afterwards, in March 1989, Roger Woodward joined us as our first TIGI rep. An ex-area manager from Clynol, he was a very reliable and experienced salesman. Previously he had worked as a car salesman. The idea was that he would take over all my loyal mail-order clients, whom Maria and I used to sell to. We had built up an income of about £10,000 a month worth of business and I wanted him to expand this and to manage a sales team. I thought he was the right person because he had been an area manager and he was also a professional salesman with a view to developing his career. It was an instant success and shortly afterwards we moved from Chelsea Wharf, which, as I mentioned earlier, had been awkward to run a business from. We still had no parking spaces there and the situation had become so difficult that we could not even stop to drop off deliveries or collections without getting a ticket. It became impossible to go on running a distribution company there.

I was very impressed when I went to see a potential new home for us in Brentford, late in 1988. It was massive compared to Chelsea, with 2,400 square feet of warehousing space and 1,200 square feet of offices with their own access and staircases. Best of all, there were twelve parking spots. The place was solid as a rock. It had boilers, toilets and was fully equipped. There was even lots of pleasant open space. It was lovely. The owners wanted £260,000. I thought the land alone would be worth £100,000 to £150,000. I went, 'Yes, I'm going to buy it.' We started getting the paperwork ready. Warren Toms was running the warehouse then – he is still very active in my business today. He was a strong support to me, but it was a far from simple purchase.

Three weeks later the agents phoned up to say: 'Unfortunately it's gone up to £290,000.' Warren advised me that we had to do the deal quickly but that was not easy and the price kept rising almost every day. In the end we settled for paying £365,000 and even then I had to rush the money through to complete the contract. But I was so, so happy, because I knew the facilities at Brentford created the structure.

Roger Woodward was an excellent salesman and he ran everything very well under my control – he still works with me today. We were so excited to move to Brentford to a new warehouse and Simon Cooper joined us from Chelsea Wharf to look after the stock. I said to Roger: 'You've got about £12,000 worth of business here. I'm very ambitious. What I would like you to do is to go and see all the clients and then, when you have got enough money to pay your wages, you can move up to the next level. Then I want you to hire a second rep. You give him your job and you go and get another lot of clients and move up another notch. Put another rep in your area and go and do it again. When you have got enough reps then you can manage them and build a proper structure.' He did the first lot and then hired the second lot, and he built a good team. You really need a lot of money so I started using the Toni & Guy money to build the TIGI structure – that really started us growing.

We were ready to really kick-start the rapid expansion of TIGI in the UK and worldwide. Firstly, I started a business proposition with my cousin, Francesco Celotto, who had spent time in London with us and now had his own business in southern Italy. He introduced me to his cousin, Emilio Celotto, to promote and distribute TIGI in Italy. I was as supportive as possible, and I invested a lot of money into this because I wanted so much for Italy to succeed. After a short time, however, Francesco realised that he could make more money being a hairdresser, but his cousin Emilio, who already had a distribution company supplying restaurants, decided to carry on with with distributing TIGI. We formed a joint venture company and called it TIGI Italia Srl. I worked out a new system to make us more competitive with the bigger companies so that it could buy the products directly from the manufacturer at the same cost as we were paying in the UK and instead of buying the products at a distributor's price, they would pay 5 per cent royalty on turnover, therefore we would be extremely competitive and give good value for money to our clients. We grew very quickly and Emilio was a highly ambitious and competent leader. I spent many days giving him and his team lots of advice and motivation.

Meanwhile, Francesco was very unhappy and complained to my

aunt that I had given the job to his cousin instead of him, which was a total lie. He told me his cousin would not do things very well, that he would collapse under the pressure and that he was a cheat and a twister. In fact Emilio did so well that he was making a profit selling our products in Italy, unlike in the UK, where we were not making a profit at all. I was surprised, but Italy is highly commercial and he could charge a bit more. In Britain the price is very important to people.

We developed TIGI in Italy with the strong support, education and image of Toni & Guy so that the Italian hairdressers would benefit, making them better and more productive hairdressers with the Toni & Guy education. It was a tremendous success, grew very quickly, and became highly profitable. I spent lots of time with Emilio, introducing him to the CEOs of the major manufacturing companies and also furniture companies in northern Italy, where all the manufacturers were positioned. It was a tremendous chance for him and helped him to gain his true identity. I have to say he grabbed the opportunity with open hands.

We were greatly assisted by the introduction of Robin Powell, an incredible operator who had worked with many blue-chip companies and was a walking directory of contacts. Robin introduced the right contact in Germany: a Mr Erhard Glaser, who was a managing director of an American company. He quickly joined us and we formed TIGI Germany, following the same structure as TIGI Italy. Erhard Glaser had 15 per cent of the shares and TIGI Germany grew as fast as TIGI Italy and generated even stronger profits. Robin was soon followed by the introduction of Alan Curtis from Australia. He was retiring as a managing director and wanted to put some of his own money into running his own company so he invested in TIGI Australia. A very experienced and knowledgeable operator, he had been the president of a huge blue-chip company. He was trustworthy and confident and again followed the same structure to make these companies highly competitive and again the businesses grew very quickly and they all benefited from the strong Toni & Guy education as part of the total concept.

As we started these TIGI companies we also had Toni & Guy in the corresponding countries to support TIGI with strong local Toni & Guy education. This was especially true in Australia, where there was Toni & Guy Australia run by Dennis Langford, a very artistic and professional hairdresser and leader. Sergio Carlucci, who had previously worked closely with me for many years in Sloane Square, ran Toni & Guy Italy. Meanwhile, Toni & Guy Germany was run by Nico Pulia, an extremely sharp and astute businessman and confident teacher; also a very artistic hairdresser. He was part of Toni & Guy Germany but also had investment in TIGI Germany.

There were continuous challenges in Germany between Toni & Guy and TIGI, and of course sometimes there was a sense of conflict of interest and eventually Nico Pulia decided to concentrate on Toni & Guy while Erhard Glaser concentrated on TIGI, but it was never easy to have the two parties work together. It was some of the most challenging aspects of my job to make them work together. Sometimes in these countries strong and determined characters are what you need, but it's almost impossible to have two Italians, two Germans or two Australians working happily together. In fact, it has become a recurring problem to try and make, for example, two Koreans or two Japanese work together – it seems you never stop learning and always have to be prepared to start again.

★ ★ ★

A brilliant young hairdresser from Japan arrived in my life in 1974 and became an important member of the Toni & Guy family. I will always be grateful to Kenji Saiga, who came to London and was extremely influential in the growth of Toni & Guy. From the start he was extremely professional and participated in the very first shows with Toni & Guy, back in the seventies. He was a highly talented guy, who became an artistic director and did wonderful work for us. I was very sad and disappointed when Kenji decided to go back to Japan in 1984.

He made the difficult decision because his son Hide, who had been born in the UK, was approaching six years old and he wanted him to be educated in the Japanese culture. I know Kenji would have loved to stay in London, but he felt that he had to go back for the benefit of his family. He was a great employee and I did not want to lose him so it was at that point that I encouraged him to open a Toni & Guy salon in Japan. There was one major problem: he didn't have any capital.

I never like to be beaten when I have an idea and I remember saying to him at the time: 'As long as you've got good health, we can find the money.' I was keen to help him as much as I could and I told him that he could take with him lots of videos, books, posters, bags, wallets… literally everything bearing the Toni & Guy logo (all these Toni & Guy accessories were in great demand in Japan). I also told him that he could do seminars using the Toni & Guy name as he had been an artistic director for nearly ten years and there was a tremendous demand for Toni & Guy education. With our support and backing and these sales I was sure that he would make enough money to open his Toni & Guy salon. And he did just that.

At the same time as Bruno was in America opening the first salon in Dallas in Sherry Lane in 1985, Kenji Saiga was opening the first salon in Tokyo, Japan. It was a year after he had gone back to Japan and he opened his salon with Mascolo Ltd having 10 per cent of the shares. This was the first of many salons. Kenji was a great artist and an excellent businessman who was very honourable and loyal to Toni & Guy. Loved by all hairdressers, he projected a relaxed and calm persona and was equally loved by all his clients for being a very special artist who cherished hairdressing deeply. He was extremely ambitious and wanted to grow a big empire in Japan. I visited him regularly at the end of the eighties and early nineties. He came frequently to London – at least every year – and we had a fantastic relationship.

Our two families were very close t and we both wanted the success of Toni & Guy. He met his wife in London, though strangely enough she came from the same small village in Japan as he did. They got married soon after he met her, and he was a loving husband with three children: two boys and a girl. I recall clearly visiting Japan in 1995, and happily remember cooking an Italian dish of pasta with tomato sauce in Kenji's home in Tokyo for all the family. A young apprentice helped me carry all the groceries when we visited the local supermarket. I never imagined that I would find the best virgin olive oil from Italy, the finest tomatoes from San Marzano, spaghetti from Gragnano and original garlic, the best of the best! Who would have thought that you could buy the best products in those days as far away as Japan? I made the greatest spaghetti ever!

I returned in 1996 and 1997 (by which time his son Hide had come back to work with us in London), and many other times to support Kenji. I wanted to give him as much help and motivation as I could. It was a real pleasure every time I was in Japan and always a tremendous experience for me. Kenji was the perfect host, welcoming at all times. I loved visiting him in Japan. Kenji was quickly followed by other international Toni & Guys across the globe but we will always regard him as the first international Master Franchisee, and were deeply saddened by his death in October 2012.

CHAPTER SIXTEEN

IF YOU'VE GOT TO MAKE A MISTAKE, MAKE YOUR OWN MISTAKE

TIGI kept expanding internationally and was becoming recognised everywhere in the world as the most professional product line for hairdressers, which benefited greatly from the strong education of Toni & Guy. We could see an amazing future and now had more than forty distributors in Europe, Asia and Australia, as well as national distribution in the United Kingdom. Customers liked the fact TIGI was the only brand used by Toni & Guy. The TIGI range was made up of highly innovative hair products, and anybody who wanted to recreate the latest collections had to use them to get the right result. It became a powerful new philosophy, which gave great strength and underpinned the reputation of our entire business.

We were growing so fast that I decided to split the company into two. One part was in West Drayton, which was the warehouse and offices for TIGI, and would look after the distribution to third-party hairdressers and all of the export to other countries.

This would allow them to concentrate on cultivating the business globally and be more attentive to details and give the best possible service at the same time, bringing in new products and also concentrating on packaging.

I remember very clearly the first board meeting when the first financial director, Terry Bellamy, was looking to get a new modern warehouse to provide a better image for the company at a rental of around £120,000 a year. Previously I had bought a freehold in Brentford and later Feltham because my insecurity as a child continued to force me towards building a strong defence and security for the company and my family.

An opportunity came our way in the shape of a repossession from Barclays. It was a freehold warehouse for sale in West Drayton, comprising some 26,000 square feet of warehouse and offices and it was a few hundred yards from the centre of town, close to the station, for the astonishing price of £150,000. It was a real steal. But our solicitor was against it because there was no official 'Vacant Possession' even though I had already met the previous owner in the Oriel coffee bar next door to our salon in Sloane Square for a cappuccino and a reassuring chat about some of the history of the warehouse. If it had been sublet or if there were any leases between any parties, he would have known. He was very helpful and said I could have all the documents and leases and anything relating to the warehouse and anything that he possessed that was kept in the safe in his house, explaining that there had been one short lease for a few years for a small part of the building and it had expired a long time ago. There was no lease active at the moment, he assured me. He wished me luck and was sorry that the business hadn't worked for him. To be totally sure of my decision I offered him compensation for his troubles and documents and he responded: 'I have already had my delicious cappuccino,' wished me good luck and left.

A few days later I called a board meeting to make a decision on the purchase of the West Drayton warehouse, which I felt could be a great buy. My lawyer, all the managers and all the heads of departments were present, including my accountant, who was never wrong. He was 100 per cent sure that we should get a new lease for fifteen years without a break at a rent of £120,000 rather than purchasing a freehold that needed some refurbishment for £150,000. I wanted to be sure that I would make the right decision, so although I felt that this would be a good buy I accepted that after all I was not a legal person and neither was I a totally qualified accountant, however my gut feeling was telling me to buy the property.

So I asked direct questions to the lawyer and he responded that he didn't feel I should go ahead with the purchase because there could be problems with no vacant possession. I asked if it would still be my freehold and he said yes, but warned that if I spent money doing it up then someone could come from nowhere and present me with a lease, which might mean that they would occupy it for that length of time. I then asked the same question of the accountant and he directly told me that he was 100 per cent sure that it would be better for the company to take a new warehouse with a 15-year lease at the rental of £120,000 and this would be deducted from the future profits and that was his recommendation. There was a bit of silence and then I suddenly remembered something my father had told me years before: 'If you have got to make a mistake, make your own mistake. Then at least you'll learn from it.'

Suddenly I felt six foot tall and sure of my decision so without being rude I banged my fist on the table and told them that I had made my decision and I wanted to go ahead and purchase the freehold. To my total astonishment the lawyer said, 'Fantastic, what a great buy you are making!' He said: 'Go ahead.' And he was supported by the full board. They were right – six months later I was offered close to £3,000,000 for the same place. This was another great lesson learned on my journey: if you take someone else's decision you will be responsible for their mistakes without learning anything.

I then created a new holding company called Cast Limited. The name came from our family initials: C for Christian, A for Anthony, S for Sacha and T for Toni. I also established a trading company called Innovia Limited at our new warehouse in Langley to concentrate solely on distributing TIGI products to Toni & Guy salons and franchises in the UK and throughout the world. Straight Impact was also born. It was a business that specialised in everything from shop fitting to selling a range of hairdressing furniture plus electrical fittings, equipment and tiles. These would be sold in all our Toni & Guy salons and third party hairdressers. Innovia had a full range of accessories and any products from coffee, disinfectant and pharmaceuticals to teabags and overalls products needed by the Toni & Guy chain of salons.

Innovia was the company that would distribute TIGI products, and become a one-stop shop. For example, Innovia sold all the TIGI products and some tints, some bleach, some peroxide. It started before the demerger and then we would take care of the salons, to help the salons get the best value. Innovia would supply everything: from light bulbs and toilet paper to everyday essentials like disinfectant, coffee and tea. If you went to the little shops in Mayfair for all these items they tended to cost a lot of money.

Innovia could supply anything the salons needed as cheaply as possible. Sometimes I would look in the petty cash at a salon and find someone had bought plasters from the local chemist and I would say to them: 'You keep them yourself.' I tried to drill into the heads of all our staff that the most important thing was to always get all of the supplies from Innovia and then we could save money.

During my many visits to Australia I had seen for myself the considerable benefits of having an efficient computer system. I realised this was something which would help us greatly so I formed a computer system which became an instant success and also helped the growth of Toni & Guy immensely. This was later made available to third-party companies, where it was similarly beneficial. It is called SalonGenius. The whole set-up in Langley, where we had moved from the previous warehouse in Feltham, became a very profitable business venture and I relied immensely on the help of my first apprentice, who later became my first PA, Maria Carabine. She was the same girl who helped me bag thousands of TIGI rollers and colour gels, some ten or twelve years earlier, and came back to join me.

Maria helped me set up a highly efficient distribution company and later on we were joined by Sally Seuke, who had some experience in distribution. Sally became a rock to me. She was very motivated and hard-working and so determined she seemed to have something to prove to herself. She was an excellent employee, extremely loyal and supportive to me, and she followed my vision. Together we grew into a large business.

Now I really believed we had a team to distribute efficiently and quickly to all Toni & Guy salons. We constantly researched new products and accessories, anything to save money for the ever-growing Toni & Guy and Essensuals Empire. We also made a very good profit while TIGI Ltd concentrated on developing third-party exports with a professional team of salesmen and experienced managers.

Sally quickly became a highly valued member of the Toni & Guy family. I became extremely fond of her and trusted her totally; she stayed with me for a long time. I was planning to further build on our success with her help and open a cash-and-carry for third-party hairdressers – I thought it would be very successful with all the experience that we had in supplying hundreds of Toni & Guy & Essensuals salons. Sally could have gone into that role and would have managed the new ideas.

After the Toni & Guy and Toni & Guy USA demerger in 2002 (to be discussed later), I was forced to start a new professional product line and needed an experienced salesman to manage and develop a sales force and create a new product line. This was a must so I could support my academies with a flow of students from all over the world. After the demerger TIGI Global now owned by my brothers had changed their policy on selling TIGI products to hairdressers supported by Toni & Guy education and had moved it to commercial advertising in magazines as they felt this would be a better way for them. Sadly, this resulted in a lack of students coming to the Toni & Guy Academy. I was confident that it would be a new era of growth, on one hand through a product company and the distribution of products, and on another by having a one-stop shop where we could supply all our Toni & Guy salons and help them to grow by offering them the best possible price. Unfortunately following the arrival of the product manager in 2005, Sally seemed to lose confidence despite continuous assurances from me not to worry about anybody else and to concentrate on her future and that her job was not only safe, we could also continue to grow and she too could grow with the company and take more responsibility.

There were two clearly separate parts of the business not conflicting with one and other, and each could grow tremendously. I made this statement very clear on many occasions but Sally was determined to leave. For me it was a sad day because I had tried everything in my power to persuade her to stay and it was a great disappointment; I felt that I had failed to manage the situation correctly. I will always miss Sally and always remember her for her contribution to the success of Toni & Guy and Innovia.

CHAPTER SEVENTEEN

SACHA AND ESSENSUALS

Both Toni & Guy and TIGI were growing at an incredible rate throughout the 1990s. The atmosphere was buoyant and everybody in the company was totally motivated and confident about the future. It really seemed that the bigger it grew, the closer the family of Toni & Guy became. Everyone was excited to be part of this fantastic dream. I believe we all knew we were creating something that was unique, the first organisation of its kind in the world, and we felt privileged to be a part of it.

By the end of 1996 we had opened thirty-one more Toni & Guy salons in the UK and by this time we were an established one-stop shop providing image and education with a strong Artistic Team in Academies. We had step-by-step videotapes and hair books and all kinds of accessories, from T-shirts, combs, scissors and hairdryers to a full range of TIGI hair products. Through our new company, Straight Impact, we also offered a full range of furniture, provided shopfitting at manufacturers' prices and had created our own computer system, Salon Genius. We offered a complete accountancy service and were fully prepared with a full team of franchise managers to support all the franchisees' needs.

Also in 1996 we opened our first salons in Germany, Sweden, Holland, Australia and Italy. In 1997 we opened twenty-one more Toni & Guy salons and also started our new sister company of hair salons, Essensuals, which was run by my daughter Sacha. It was the right time to create something of her own, to put her own creative feelings and ideas into something, and to come away from the shadow of my brother Anthony. I wanted her to be more herself and to show her own talent and have her own company, as Anthony wanted to keep all of his shares in Toni & Guy. So it was my wish and duty to give her this opportunity and my God, did she excel!

Sacha created an incredible image, which was fresh and exhilarating. It was the fastest-growing hairdressing chain that ever opened: fifty salons were opened in just over two years. This became a great opportunity for all Toni & Guy franchisees to expand to a second salon in the same city.

I always hoped that Sacha would play a leading role in the business, but in my wildest imagination I could not have dreamt how fantastic she would be by my side. Of course I am hopelessly biased because she is my only daughter, but Sacha has helped to turn us into what we are today. I'd like her to explain a little of our relationship herself.

Sacha says:

My father Toni has dedicated his whole life to the family, to all of us. He is the most unselfish person in the world. He doesn't like buying clothes, he doesn't like spending money and he's not bothered about having a fast car. My mother, on the other hand, does like buying clothes! They're like complete opposites. Actually without my mum I don't think my dad would have made so much money because she loves to spend it.

I always thought you had to be ruthless and harsh to be a top businessman and he's shown me that you don't. My dad is an amazing businessman and the complete opposite of that. He taught me that someone else's success can be your success. If you help other people to grow then you can grow. He is so kind, he hates to hurt anyone, but then he is also the best businessman that I know. He would always say, 'Don't think about the money, just love what you do, then the money will come.' He is very humble and down to earth. He doesn't like spending money so he goes on the train to work; he doesn't like getting a cab if the Tube can get you there cheaper.

He is exactly the same as he was before he had money – he could live in a small house quite happily. He does everything for the family. He could take life much easier and really spoil himself and that would make me feel happy. Instead as soon as he gets some money he'll say, 'Well, I've put that money into investments so that when I've gone, it'll be there for you.' I say, 'Just spend it yourself.' He loves to work so hard and he really doesn't like spending money. We have such a great relationship. I can go into any meeting and feel so much better because he is there. I have learned so much from him, and I am still learning all the time.

Essensuals was born and certainly made its mark with Sacha working quite brilliantly at the helm. She exceeded all my expectations as she drove the company to success after success. Toni & Guy continued with its expansion in the UK by opening a further twenty-nine salons in 1998, along with twenty more Essensuals salons and ten overseas Toni & Guy salons. That seemed remarkable but 1999 was even more unbelievable as the expansion went on. Even today I find it hard to understand how that was achieved. I opened an amazing thirty Toni & Guy salons, while Sacha opened twenty-two Essensuals salons, and we also opened over twenty overseas salons. It was fantastic! We saw the first salons open in Cyprus, Singapore, Norway, Greece, Malta, Ireland and France. As we started to expand worldwide I felt so proud – it was as if I was walking on air. It was such an amazing feeling of satisfaction and happiness to be able to give so much opportunity and success to these young artists, who were excited and very willing hairdressers who trusted me to help them achieve their dreams.

Often I went back to remembering my childhood. I thought back to the days when I was this young boy of fourteen living in Italy when I could not have imagined in my wildest dreams what life had in store for me. Now, when everything was going so well for my family and me, I took time to remember when I arrived in London and was out of work for two days. I remembered being so worried and disheartened and so anxious to get a job and I compared those feelings to the happiness of success. I considered my previous position and thought about what I had achieved and I felt extremely humbled, lucky and grateful. I've always valued what I've had but most of all, respected it. And I've always tried to put myself in the place of others, of my family and my employees, to see what they would expect from me, and I tried not to disappoint them.

After all, I knew deep down in my heart that Toni & Guy's success is their success and I would be nothing without them. As d'Artagnan used to say to the three musketeers: 'All for one, one for all!' That's Toni & Guy's motto, too. It was a very exciting time because I knew we had a great formula for success and it gave me a lot of confidence. I had to find a way to pass on the same confidence to my young franchisees, some of whom had worked side by side with me as young apprentices, and I wanted to help them achieve their dreams – it was both my duty and my destiny.

Although the nineties were incredibly successful, one thing that remained with me as a moment of great sadness was the plight of my friend and mentor, Kurt Andersen. When I met him in London he confided in me some very sad news. He had discovered that his trusted accountant had stolen continuously from his company, his pride and joy, his security and his livelihood. I learned to my horror that he was in danger of losing everything. At that time he also owed my own company, TIGI Ltd., a considerable amount of money. Seeing my old friend so down and close to despair, my first reaction was to tell him not to worry. I told him getting so down was not worthy of him – 'Don't let something like this kill you. We will work together. Your debt to me is already cancelled,' I said.

I tried to lift his spirits by insisting it was only money and that I would be 100 per cent behind him. We had a strong business, I told him, and this setback was really not worth worrying about – 'We'll make it OK, please don't worry. I'm there for you and together we will win this situation.' I sincerely thought that my intervention would help get him back into the same frame of mind he was a few months earlier, full of life and good spirits and excited about the future. But tragically a few evenings later I had a call from Mrs

Andersen and she told me the terrible news that her dear husband had suffered a massive heart attack and he had left us.

It was a horrible shock and one of my saddest moments. I knew that I would miss him very much and probably forever. He was a friend and he was a colleague, someone very, very dear to me and it left a big hole in my life. It made me remember how important he had been, always giving me good advice to help me carry on. Although he was quiet, he had a huge personality and was always ready to help with manufacturing new products from our ideas and introducing me to valuable contacts and businessmen. Definitely an invaluable asset and also my best friend, he had helped me open the first Toni & Guy school in Copenhagen and had travelled regularly to Basle, where we made our first deal with a Swiss manufacturing company that was producing under licence to Eugène Perma, Paris, similar to his company in Denmark, which was one of his associates. They would manufacture and distribute TIGI products under licence to the Swiss market with a contract of royalties to Mascolo Ltd. It was a great learning process that helped me to understand different ways of distribution and export.

Mr Andersen had loved Paris – we met there regularly at every opportunity, especially when he visited Eugène Perma. Our journey together to achieve worldwide network distribution will always live in my heart forever.

★ ★ ★

Happily, there were some lighter moments in my life as the decade drew to a close. It was 13 November 1999 when I left home to go to the Bahamas, where we were to put on a show for some 700 hairdressers, most of whom were women. Sacha and Christian came along, as did my friend Nico Pulia from Germany. We stayed a week in this amazing resort hotel, in the Caribbean.

It was the perfect trip except that one of the girls was chasing after me! For me there has only ever been one woman so there was no question that she would ever have any success, but my son was annoyed and he got a little bit touchy about it. The girl in question was German and Christian sent one of his friends also German, to warn off this amorous young lady. Apparently she let rip and said: 'You disgraceful creature, you know he is a married man!' But as she said it in German I did not know what they were saying.

When I asked what the conversation was about, Christian tactfully pretended she had said that she had left a coat on the plane!

CHAPTER EIGHTEEN

A TERRIBLE DAY...
AND THE MOST
WONDERFUL DAY

I have faced a great many challenges in my life and often they have come out of nowhere, as a complete and terrifying surprise. The worst of those moments came in the summer of the year 2000 on what should have been a happy trip to my homeland of Italy. I suffered a stroke. This shocked me to the core. Even today I do not find it easy to talk about this experience. I will recount my memories of the incident and then let Pauline give her version.

I had begun the new millennium on the crest of a wave. The nineties had vanished and everyone seemed enthused about stepping into a new century. The business was doing well and life seemed full of opportunity and optimism.

As the year 2000 arrived, my mind was full of all the things I wanted to achieve. There had been discussions with my brothers about a parting of the ways. They were focused on America and everything they could do there, while I was very happy in the UK as a base for all our international operations. We had been together as brothers since the early 1960s and we would always be close as family. Now we all had children of our own and young families to take care of in the future. I was becoming more relaxed to the idea of a demerger of the business. After all we had been together for approaching forty years and had enjoyed enormous success together.

To be frank I did not have too much time to dwell on difficulties and problems, because there were so many amazing developments going on. I had never known such excitement in business growth. It was astonishing, like a boom time. Back then it seemed you could do nothing wrong – the turn of the century appeared to give the whole economy a breath of fresh air. Turnover was increasing month by month and you could plan continuous growth. As I look back now I just remember that for a blissful time it was easy, so easy. Everybody in all companies, including Toni & Guy and TIGI, was looking ahead at the start of the year 2000. No one was talking about anything else but a bright future. The celebrations were incredible for everybody, and it seemed that, like ourselves, all traders shared great hopes for the future. Even the dreaded 'Millennium Bug' failed to materialise! It was all good news.

It was fabulous to be in London for the Millennium. Prime Minister Tony Blair, who celebrated with HM the Queen and thousands of others at the Millennium Dome, said the 'confidence and optimism' of the occasion should be bottled and kept forever. More than 2,000,000 people lined the banks of the River Thames to watch a firework spectacular, while in Rome the Pope delivered a special New Year blessing, urging people to work hard to make the next 1,000 years a time of peace around the world. I agreed with them both – it felt like a special time to be alive. In New York's Times Square some four tons of confetti rained down on countless revellers, but I still felt that London was the capital of the world.

As the year 2000 finally arrived and business continued in the same frenetic rhythm I was absolutely delighted that nothing had changed except that we felt more confident than ever to start new salons, and a lot of young franchisees were confident enough to take on the challenge of running their own business. Everyone was very excited – to do business was to be alive. We opened more than twenty new Toni & Guy salons in the year 2000 in countries as varied as Dubai and Austria, and at home in the UK, in locations as different as Chesterfield and Stratford-upon-Avon. We opened quite a few Essensuals as well, as expansion was the order of the day.

On a personal level, Pauline and I were delighted that our daughter Sacha seemed to have found happiness with her boyfriend James Tarbuck, son of the famous comedian, Jimmy Tarbuck. In February 2000 we attended a wonderful party to celebrate Jimmy Tarbuck's sixtieth birthday. It was a glittering occasion and there were many famous show business and sporting faces there. I enjoyed talking with the football star Kevin Keegan very much, though I was a bit embarrassed to admit to him that Pauline hates football. He laughed and said his wife hated it as well! He was with Alan Hansen, often seen on the BBC's *Match of the Day* as a respected pundit (and recently retired in 2014), and I made a bit of a boob. I wanted to pay him a compliment but I became a little muddled: I told him that my friend, Gianfranco Zola, had said to me that he was the best centre-back he had faced when he played against England. Hansen smiled and said: 'Toni, Toni, Toni, you are lying! I am *not* English, I am Scottish!' It was an awkward moment. I was very embarrassed and said I must have got confused. That's what happens when you tell a white lie – it backfires!

Then, later in 2000, we created Zoya, a wonderful new shop that was born of Pauline's own brilliant vision. It was back in the days when the Body Shop was very successful and she had spotted another potential gap in the market. Like so many good ideas, it was extremely simple: it was for there to be a shop where you could buy that special present, something stylish and out of the ordinary. It was Pauline's idea, but of course I wanted to help make it a success so I got involved. We planned to open the first shop in Kingston, and Pauline found suitable premises and then carefully put together an exciting selection of products, from perfume to jewellery and lots of other things as well. She threw herself into all the planning and organising. And when my wife throws herself into something she really is whole-hearted – you'd better not get in her way!

Of course I very much wanted to contribute and I was eager to do something for men so I suggested that we should go to Italy to find some really elegant and exclusive products that were not available in other English stores. In August 2000, with our friend Emilio, Pauline and I flew to my home country to take a look at this special exhibition. We were hunting for some new and exclusive items, such as ties that you couldn't buy anywhere else or some original shirts. Pauline has a very good eye for what will appeal and I was anxious to support her as much as possible. It was a shop for people who wanted to buy really special presents, perhaps a wife shopping for her husband or the other way round. And all the gifts were to be very beautifully wrapped, and Pauline insisted all the cards the shop sold must be elegant and handmade.

The exhibition was to be staged in Puglia (or Apulia, as it is called in English), in the south-east. As we drove across from Sorrento on the west coast where we were staying with friends, I began to feel very strange and unwell. I tried to shake off the sensation but as the journey went on it gradually grew worse and worse. We stopped at a garage on the way and I was feeling a bit uneasy and uncomfortable. Although I was in my own country, the Italy that I love, somehow I did not feel at all at home: things seemed to have changed for the worse in ways I could not quite put my finger on. It should have been a supremely happy experience, travelling with Pauline and working together on her exciting new enterprise, but for me it was the complete opposite. I felt uneasy, unwell and unhappy – all in all, terrible.

We were quite near Apulia when we stopped to get some petrol. I went inside to get a cup of coffee (I love coffee and I thought that it might make me feel better). I still felt very strange as I went back towards the car. It was a very odd experience – I could walk and talk, but I did not feel right. Pauline screamed as soon as she saw me – she saw that my face had dropped and realised what was happening. She wanted help, and she shouted so loudly she got it. She got ambulances, she got the fire brigade, and she got the police! I think all Italy must have known what was happening. At first I still did not want any fuss – I was trying to say I was all right. I was asking for another cappuccino, and Pauline was panicking.

Everybody rushed around and took me to the hospital. And the doctor there took one look at me and said straight away: 'You have had a stroke so we will have to hospitalise you.' I didn't like that at all so I said: 'No, I don't want to stay here.' I remember getting up to walk out, and I remember going back to Sorrento.

As it turned out, I was very lucky. When I had the stroke, my face had dropped, but fortunately for me the blood was still getting through to the brain. The doctor explained afterwards that my brain had been unaffected. I really only suffered a lack of blood, which was certainly a shock to the system. Later, when I saw the specialist, he said if it had been a year earlier they would have operated on me. He explained that they used to operate on everybody who had my kind of stroke in order to unblock the arteries near the brain. And he said in 98 per cent of cases the patient died. I was stunned to learn that only two in one hundred survived. This was because the surgery was so close to the most sensitive parts of the brain, the doctor explained, and said they had stopped performing that particular operation because they found it was unnecessary as usually the blood finds a different way to get to the brain.

To be honest, I know that Pauline's memory of this very frightening incident in my life is much better than mine so I will let her explain.

Pauline says:

This was a difficult time for Toni because there had already been some talk between him and his brothers over demerging the business. Toni was under even more pressure than ever, but of course pressure was something I had watched him thrive under for years and years.

Zoya was my dream, but Toni wanted to be involved and it was wonderful to be working closely with him again. I'd had the Kingston salon franchised out and because all my children had gone off, I wanted to do something with my life. I had always wanted to have a shop where people could buy those really special presents. When it came to customers I was thinking particularly of men, who are not always great at thinking of the perfect gift. I wanted to give them a choice of lovely things, and then, after they had made their selection, to have their present all beautifully wrapped. It would be so simple. All they had to do was listen to a little good advice and they could walk out and it would all be done. I was full of enthusiasm for the new project and of course I also wanted to sell TIGI products. Toni agreed it was a good idea and was keen to support me all the way.

We found a shop in a great location and worked hard to get everything ready. The lease was waiting to be signed. Everything was ready and absolutely perfect and because we wanted the very best and to be different, Toni and I decided we would go to Italy to source some really stunning stock. I wanted lovely things, like the stylish Italian clothing and products you didn't find in England in those days. We were looking for a whole range of things from shirts, ties and jumpers to cufflinks, gloves and other items, all designed in Italy.

This was all happening at about the time the brothers were talking about demerging the business. It was a complex and very personal problem that needed to be solved. Toni had all that on his mind. I was concerned that I was adding to his load of responsibilities by accepting his help in setting up Zoya, but he said: 'No, it's great. If we do the demerger then it's good for you to have something of your own.' We went to Italy, where there was a big exhibition for buyers. I was very excited and looking forward to it a lot. We were staying in a hotel in Sorrento and a friend of ours who was in TIGI decided to come as well. We were on the road early in the morning as it was a long way – we had to drive right across Italy.

It turned into a terrible day that I will never forget because that was when Toni had his stroke. We had stopped off to buy some petrol. Toni had been to the toilet and we were in the car, waiting for him to come out. I realised as soon as I saw him walking back towards the car that he had had a stroke. He looked white, ashen even. His face had dropped a little bit and he wasn't focusing on anything. I just started to scream for help. Toni was looking at me and he kept saying he was all right but I knew he wasn't and I got him to admit that he didn't feel 'all that well'.

As luck would have it, two policemen were in this filling station and they came over. I said: 'My husband's having a stroke. I know he is. He's got to get to a hospital as soon as possible.' They got the ambulance to come within minutes and then they gave us an escort to the hospital. They were absolutely wonderful; in fact, everyone seemed to really want to help us. They rushed him in and checked him out and confirmed my feeling that it was a stroke. They said that I had got him there just in time and they put him on drips and everything else and thankfully enough the next morning, when he woke up, he wasn't paralysed. It was amazing! He just looked very unwell. They wanted him to stay in the hospital, but he wanted to come home.

He was definitely not allowed to fly, but he was still determined to come home as soon as possible. He desperately wanted to be with the children – it was the most important thing in the world to him. We thought about a car or a train, but the journey seemed as if it would be too much for him. He didn't want to stay in the hospital in Puglia. We were in shock and a long, long way from home and not really sure what to do for the best. Eventually I persuaded the doctor to let him go back to Sorrento. She reluctantly said: 'OK, but first we will do as many stress tests as we can here. He can't fly yet, but in a week, maybe.' She said it was OK to drive Toni in the car back to Sorrento but she was very firm and insisted: 'He must not do anything, and I really mean *anything*.'

It was much better back in Sorrento, where we had friends and family, but it was still horrible because I couldn't do anything for him – I couldn't leave him for a second. We went to a specialist, who said Toni must stay there until the end of the week at least. They had a wheelchair waiting for him and they were adamant that he had to have complete rest; he was not even allowed to walk. It was very frustrating and frightening. Toni hated being cooped up and it was worse being away from home. The fact we were so far away from our children made everything much more difficult for both of us. I was horrified to even think of life without Toni, and he was struggling to cope with the stroke.

I think it was the worst time of our lives. We talked to the children on the telephone a lot and of course they wanted to rush out to Italy to be with us but there was no point as we were going home. They were all very, very upset. We did eventually get home at the end of a desperately long week that seemed like an age, and the three children were all naturally very emotional. They were delighted to see their father back home, but very concerned about what he had been through and about his chances of making a full recovery. We have always been very close but you never forget experiences like that and of course it brought us even closer together as a family. It was an ordeal for all of us that none of us would want to go through again. Fortunately, our older son Christian stepped up to lead us all through this terrible time – he was a real brick. He supported me and his father and his brother and sister. He surprised me with his strength and I was very proud of him.

The impact of Toni's stroke was felt far and wide. News travels fast in any close-knit society and everyone knows everyone in our business. Even far-flung Toni & Guy outposts all over the world were soon anxiously asking for updates on Toni's health. To be honest, everybody in the business was absolutely terrified. There was no huge management team to take over the enormous responsibility of running our large and complex organisation. Toni is Toni & Guy – and he always has been. It has always been hard for people to understand how one man controls so much but my husband has never been an ordinary businessman. Right from the start, it all went on in his head – the planning, the strategy, the decisions – and since Toni & Guy started, back in 1963, it had always worked wonderfully well. Of course he has lots of advisers, managers, accountants, lawyers and what-have-you, but essentially, Toni had always been the driving force. Everything went on inside his head. I don't know how one man managed it, but he did. And of course he had always done it very successfully, too.

Yet now the great strength of Toni & Guy was suddenly turned into an alarming potential weakness. As the news about Toni's stroke spread, I realised that everyone was running scared. So many people relied on him for leadership and direction that now he was no longer there we had to do something quickly to reassure them all that it really was business as usual. I told Christian that we had to take over his father's role. Initially I said to him: 'Get them all to come to me.' I took all the phone calls and Christian and I dealt with everything. It worked, and I like to think that we steadied the ship at a very awkward time. But getting Toni back into action was another matter.

My husband is the most positive person I know. For years I had watched him handle a massive workload with amazing energy and enthusiasm. I know that I am biased, but he is a remarkable man. Yet after his stroke, Toni was not at all himself. For the first time in his life he got a bit depressed. I think the stroke was a real shock for him mentally, as well as a setback physically, and he did not recover straight away.

He was at home for six weeks and I could see he was really struggling. Although his body seemed to be getting better, his mind was clearly still very troubled. As I did my best to care for him, never wanting to leave his side for long, I realised that springing back into action was really difficult for him. It seemed as though he didn't want to do anything. It almost felt as if he did not want to live any more. He even missed our big occasion at the Royal Albert Hall on 24 September. It was the first time we had put on a big show without him. Toni told me later he was very frightened. It was a truly awful time, mostly for him, but also for the whole family, who love him so much.

I have always believed in taking direct action when it is necessary and I decided to tackle the situation head-on. One morning I confronted him and I said, 'Right, I have had enough of this behaviour! There is no point in me living any longer if you are not back with me the way you used to be.' He looked shocked as I went on, 'You need to get back to your old self and do something like you used to do. I can't bear to watch you like this a moment longer.' The very next day he got up early, like he always did before the stroke, and showered and went back to the office. Of course he was not his old self instantly. It took time, but it started that day. Gradually he got stronger and stronger and, thankfully, soon I had my old Toni back.

I could not have been happier. It was awful to have to speak so harshly to the man I love, but I had to do it to save him. I wanted the old Toni back and I was so happy when that is what I got. I think that from outside it looks as if we have everything, thanks to Toni's success. We are very fortunate financially, of course, and money gives you a lovely life, but when a situation like Toni's stroke hits a family, wealth means absolutely nothing. People are much more important than possessions. That is something Toni and I have always agreed upon.

Gradually Toni's health recovered but by then I found that my heart was no longer in the shop. Zoya started as a dream but it ended for me in the nightmare of my husband's illness. After the stroke I couldn't leave Toni for quite a while so I gave up all thoughts of running the shop myself. I got a manager in to run the place. I had no choice but I knew in my heart that it was far from an ideal solution. I started to have my doubts about the shop. Then as Toni's health improved I did go in for a while and I started to feel Zoya might be a success in spite of everything but suddenly Toni had another serious health problem.

He was in a lot of pain and it turned out he needed an operation for gallstones. It felt as though everything was coming down on us one after another. Evidently he'd had them for years and not known. That was pretty bad for him. He had a lot of pain and I was looking after him pretty much full-time again. I was changing dressings and doing all sorts of things so again I had to rely on a manager to look after Zoya. That turned out to be a bad idea: when I studied the figures they were very poor and all of a sudden the shop was not doing very well at all. I couldn't understand it because previously everything had been going well. The range of goods we found certainly brought in the customers and it seemed my original idea had been pretty good. But then a friend told me she had found the shop shut when it should have been open. When I went round to investigate I was horrified to find that I had employed a very lazy manager who really let me down. In the end Toni & Guy took it over. It taught me I wanted to be free to take care of Toni and the family.

There could never be a good time for Toni to have a stroke but it came when we were still doing up the house. The major work was nearly finished but there were still lots of jobs to do. The house was my project. I designed it, with a little help, of course, and it was very important to me to get it right. I took charge of all the work and some of the situations I got involved in were a nightmare. Once I even had to build some specially curved steps myself to show the builders exactly how I wanted them! Toni said he only ever wanted to come to it when it was completely finished so it was definitely my project.

We lived in the original bungalow that was on the site here for two and a half years while doing the plans. I really threw myself into getting our dream house to be perfect, but when Toni had his stroke I hated the house. Thank God it was just about finished apart from the outside. If anything had happened to Toni I would have sold it straight away – I wouldn't have wanted to live in it without Toni.

Of course I felt the same. I would never have wanted to live in Summerdown Manor, the house Pauline had worked so hard to make perfect for us, without her. I was determined to regain my full health in time for our daughter Sacha's wedding. Summerdown was a brand-new house, built on the site of a bungalow, which we lived in for a time. But in July 1999 we moved to a house called Casabella, in nearby Cobham, while all the work was taking place. We knocked the bungalow down, and Pauline got to work with the architects and builders on planning and building the new house. By the time of Sacha's wedding in August 2001 we had almost finished the shell of the house. From the outside it looked great, just like a fully completed house. In fact there was still a lot to do. There was no heating, no kitchen, no water – there was hardly anything, it was just a shell.

We had the wedding in the garden, and Pauline worked hard to make it look nice by putting lots of flowers all over the place, so we could come inside and take photographs. That cost me £400,000 because the VAT people said the house was completed, so we had to pay the VAT on everything. I said: 'We're still living in Casabella in Cobham!' I explained to the VAT people that this house had no heating or kitchen, but they said: 'We don't care, as far as we are concerned you were living there, in Summerdown.' Apparently the law says that when you build a new house you are exempt from VAT, but as soon as you live in it you must start paying VAT. That cost £400,000 as they just would not believe that we genuinely had not moved in.

But Sacha's wedding was such a wonderful occasion that I soon forgot about the money. I just left everything to Pauline and she can best describe how well it went.

Pauline says:

When Sacha was just two years old I remember Toni saying that he was going to start saving up to pay for her wedding. Talk about thinking ahead! But we both knew for years that it was always a most important event in our future. Toni always wanted it to be the most special day. He used to say to me: 'When she gets married she can have whatever she wants.' That was quite a statement from my husband who, despite his success, is always careful how he spends his money. He still uses the Tube and he never wants to fly first class unless I push him into it.

When Sacha started going out with James Tarbuck, son of the famous comedian Jimmy Tarbuck, we were both delighted to see her so happy. James seemed like a fine young man and Toni and I felt they were made for each other. We have both always been well aware of how lucky we were to find each other and to enjoy such a long and happy marriage so of course we wanted nothing less for our daughter. But after Toni's stroke somehow it became more and more important that the wedding happened as quickly as possible. Sacha was keen to push the date forward to 22 August 2001. It sounds a little dramatic with hindsight, considering Toni's amazing recovery to full health, but at the time we all desperately wanted to make sure that Toni was there for the big day.

As Toni said, the house was not finished, but we knew that would not matter because we could use the garden for the reception. Sacha and I got together to plan the big day. I remember I said, 'We'll get a wedding co-ordinator to help organise all the details but we will stay in total control and we will do everything together to make this the greatest wedding ever.' Sacha pointed out that we needed to sit down with Daddy and put together a budget. She said: 'We've got to know what we're looking at.' Sacha is very good with money. She is an excellent businesswoman in her own right but she was wary of her father's reaction. She knew she needed to know how much money she could spend and she said, 'He's going to say something ridiculous, that you can't buy a bean with.' In fact, Toni's response surprised me just as much as it surprised Sacha. He said: 'Whatever you want, you have it. There is not a budget. Spend as much as you need.' We were both stunned but of course I soon realised my husband had said something very shrewd as well as very generous. He knew perfectly well that both Sacha and I were very careful with money so the responsibility was ours to look for the right deals and not abuse his generosity. When I thought about it, I realised it was a very clever thing to say.

We planned the whole thing like a military operation. First things first, we wanted to get a really special dress and we decided early on that we wanted one designed by Elizabeth Emanuel. That was not so easy. She was very busy, until we explained that it was for the only daughter of Toni Mascolo, owner of Toni & Guy. I don't like using Toni's name to get favours but when it comes to your daughter's wedding dress, it's different! A message came back that Sacha could have her Emanuel dress.

After that planning the actual wedding was fun. We had lots of celebrities on our guest list because James's dad seemed to number just about every famous face in show business among his friends. They all helped to make it a special day. We wanted it to be a full-of-fun day. We wanted children among the congregation and we really wanted everyone to enjoy themselves.

The service was in Mayfair and it was a wonderful service. We stayed in the Connaught for the night before. Sacha and James had a horse and carriage to take them to the church! Then we had lots of cars bringing us back to the house for a reception for 750 people. We could have gone up to over 1,000 but you have to draw the line somewhere. We had a funfair on the lawn and we were blessed with beautiful weather. In the end it really was fun for all concerned, which was exactly what we had wanted. And organising the wedding was such fun – Sacha and I loved being in complete control. James put it best when he said dryly in his speech that he would like to thank, Pauline and Sacha for inviting him to this wedding!

It really was the most wonderful day – I think it was the hottest day for 100 years. We had lots of priests and nuns there among the guests and Toni said in his speech that he thanked them very much for their prayers for the weather, though he said considering the sunshine perhaps they had 'overdone it a little'.

CHAPTER NINETEEN

DEMERGER

Toni & Guy is first and foremost a family business. Here, please note that for me family *always* comes before business. My love for my family is what led me to start the business in the first place. Family will always be the most important thing in the world for me, but situations change as decades go by. As the year 2003 approached, my brothers and I were all well aware that we were coming up to our fortieth anniversary. It was almost four decades since Guy and myself had first started working together in our humble little hairdressing salon on Clapham Park Road in the awful aftermath of our beloved mother's tragically early death.

At that time, as the oldest son, with my father racked with inconsolable grief, it fell to me to do everything I could for the family. Nothing else mattered. More than anything, I wanted to take care of my younger brothers and I worked as hard as I possibly could to get our family business off the ground. I believe that tough beginning did much to help forge the person I have become.

Back then I used to sweep up the pins from the floor and stay up late sterilising them so we could re-use them and save money. I was doing it because I did not want to waste one single penny of our precious cash. Those days were desperately difficult and I wanted to do everything I possibly could to make our business succeed. Deep down, that uncompromising attitude has never changed in me through all the years. I felt the responsibility of taking charge of the finances weighing heavily upon my shoulders but my brothers were all younger than me and although Guy was with me through the toughest times he was more than happy to concentrate on being a great hairdresser and let me look after the books. Bruno and Anthony both worked very hard certainly, but they came into the family business a few years later when things were becoming a little easier.

Through forty years together we had many ups and downs of fortune as the business grew, on both sides of the Atlantic, but we always stayed rock solid as a family. I would do anything for my brothers and I know that each of them feels the same way. But over the years I saw much less of Bruno and Guy simply because they were in America and I was in the UK. The two areas of the company were both growing and expanding very successfully and that meant we were all busier than ever. Geography saw to it that the two halves of the business grew further and further apart but there was no big bust-up. The only rift between us was the Atlantic Ocean.

I am very proud that we kept the family concern going for those forty years. We did, of course, have a few changes over the decades. It started with Guy and myself sharing everything equally, 50–50 at the start of 1963. Then, that summer, my father came in with us and we became Francisco Mascolo and Sons. My father had 34 per cent and Guy and myself had 33 per cent each! After Father died, and Bruno and Anthony came in, I decided that the four of us brothers should each have 25 per cent. I know that I could have insisted on a bigger share as I had established the business and, with Guy's happy approval, ran the show throughout the earlier years, but I thought, *If we are family, we should share everything equally. We don't want bad feeling between us.* And I believe that thought helped to keep us together for forty years, so I am proud to have made it. It was a good decision.

To work as a family is amazing. It did have its disadvantages, of course, because we argued now and again, though we always came to a resolution. But forty years is a long time. The four of us grew up and we all had families of our own. We all developed and changed in different ways so it was inevitable that sooner or later the question of the structure of the business would come up. It was only natural that my younger brothers would want to have more control and independence at some time. It is perhaps surprising that it took them so long, I think!

I certainly did not advertise it at the time but in 2001 and 2002 my health still was not so good. There was the stroke and the gall bladder. I got back to work after both my medical problems, but I think for a time I was feeling a little down. There was also the age factor. I have always been blessed with a strong constitution and I have always had a great deal of energy and never minded working long hours, but I was no longer a young man. I think I felt aware of my mortality more than ever before and that made me increasingly concerned for the future.

The demerger was not a sudden idea. Over the years I had talked with my brothers in America many times about the future and I knew that they wanted to split the business and take over the United States for themselves. Bruno, particularly, wanted to be in control and for that you cannot blame him. He was always very ambitious and I understood perfectly well that he wanted to be in charge of his own operation – it was only natural. Bruno has many good qualities and he had worked extremely hard to build up Toni & Guy in the United States. He wanted very much to be in control of his own empire without his older brother being involved.

I understood Bruno and Guy's point of view, even if I did not perhaps 100 per cent agree with it. But what made their case stronger was that Anthony agreed with Bruno and Guy, and he wanted to go over to America to work with them. He thought that was where his future lay. Anthony had built up a terrific reputation as a top hairdresser in the UK, winning many Hairdresser of the Year Awards and a big name for himself in the process. He was the famous face who brought in lots of hairdressers, who wanted our education, and the Academy side of our business was very strong. But then Anthony became fascinated by the idea of working in America. He would go over there and come back full of stories of how wonderful everything was; he would criticise things in Great Britain and insist that the United States was the best place in the world to live and work. I listened to that for a while and then he said he had decided that he wanted to move to the United States to become a crucial part of Bruno and Guy's set-up. Who was I to stand in his way? I think he thought he had achieved as much as he could in the UK and it was about time he set about conquering America.

Somewhat reluctantly, I agreed with the demerger to please my brothers. If it had been left to me alone I think I would have left the structure as it was, but my three brothers wanted this division so I went along with it. To be fair, there was some merit in the thinking behind the split. There was certainly no argument between us. The basic difference really was that I did not want to live in America and they did. I simply went along with the majority view, thinking the two businesses could each thrive on its own. I thought we could go on from our success together to create two separate worlds. I agreed that when Anthony moved to America they could take over not just the United States, but also Canada and the whole of South America as well. Anthony persuaded me that this would give them the chance to expand Toni & Guy throughout the Americas. They took TIGI as well and I was left running Toni & Guy in the rest of the world. As I said at the time: 'Now each brother can eat what he kills!'

I agreed to the demerger for one reason, and one reason only: I wanted to keep my brothers happy.

Nothing stays the same forever in life and we had enjoyed nearly forty years together in the same business. Perhaps it was time for a change, I told myself. At this time my daughter Sacha was making an extraordinary success of Essensuals. She was still very young but she built up a chain of more than sixty salons in two years. It was an almost unbelievable rate of growth and I could see that she was going to have a very big future in the business. She created a fantastic image and the salons were excellent – almost as good as Toni & Guy, I had to admit. I was very, very proud of her.

We did the demerger in 2002 and soon afterwards Anthony dropped a bombshell: he had changed his mind about going to America, for 'family reasons', and intended to stay in the UK. That meant the end of his plans to build the Academy in New York. Anthony is my brother and I love him but this did make life very difficult for me for a while. After the demerger, because of his fame and great qualities as a hairdresser, Anthony continued to do very well in the UK and he and my other brothers changed their emphasis from education to direct advertising. That meant there were fewer students who wanted to come through the Academy and at the same time I had lost Anthony, who had become a big draw for Toni & Guy. This left a big void in Toni & Guy and gave me perhaps my most challenging time in all the years of being in business.

Things were difficult for a while but this is where my daughter Sacha came in and gave my business a tremendous boost. She and Anthony were always very close and still are to this day. She herself is a brilliant stylist who won awards and had built up a big reputation of her own. I was always well aware of my own qualities – I was good at business but lacking on the artistic side. Sacha won the London Hairdresser of the Year title in the year 2000 and I was tremendously pleased for her. I always knew my daughter was very talented so it was wonderful to see her talent recognised.

Without my brothers I had to get Sacha fully involved with me at Toni & Guy and so we had to leave Essensuals in the hands of Christian for a while. It was a difficult time for us because she had to work extremely hard to replace the artistic and charismatic leadership of Anthony. Finding someone to take over from an artist of Anthony's calibre was a huge problem but Sacha solved it sensationally well. She was so passionate that she surprised us all; she was absolutely fantastic and she did it! Soon, I knew that with Sacha by my side we could be more successful than ever. Sacha was my saviour. I realise now that Anthony was getting a little older by this time and I think he was beginning to want to relax a little. Sacha had so much talent that was not being shown and this brought out that talent and allowed it to blossom.

Sacha says:

I don't know about being a saviour – I'm just doing what I love, working with my dad. He is all about family and I have such an amazing relationship with him. I absolutely adore him. He is a real inspiration and he has got the kindest heart and he is the most generous man I know. He is so kind.

We often know exactly what the other is thinking and we tend to react the same way to things. We are quite similar to each other out of everyone in the family. My mum says, 'Oh God, you're just like your dad!' We are both Taureans so I suppose that helps. But then he is business and I'm creative – that's why it works.'

CHAPTER TWENTY

WE'VE ONLY
JUST BEGUN

The early years of the new century were a time of great change and development for Toni & Guy. For all of us the demerger was a very strange experience. In one way it changed everything, in that I was now running a business completely apart from my brothers. Yet, in another way it changed nothing in that our feelings for each other as a family were as strong as ever. Happily, I felt that second emotion very strongly in 2003 when we celebrated the fortieth anniversary of the company with a memorable family party at the Grosvenor House hotel. It was wonderful to experience that remarkable landmark as part of a warm and loving family and I know my brothers felt the same way.

Deep down, as I have said, I did not want a demerger but I bowed to the majority. And once the decision had been made I did my level best to make everything work. I let Canada and South America go into my brothers' area so that they could grow their side of the business to the maximum. But Anthony's decision to stay in Britain changed many things for me. His wife had decided that she did not want to move to America after all, and that was that. It meant that Anthony's plans to open a big Academy in New York were abruptly cancelled. I had indicated that I would be happy to participate with him in that scheme, but he said: 'No, no, no! I want to do that on my own.' Then he changed his mind altogether and came to London and decided that London was the place to open their TIGI Academy because it was better for the brand. That was fine for them but it certainly took a lot of potential students out of my schools, which soon suffered and looked for a time as if they might not survive.

After Anthony opened his TIGI Academy, he obviously had to expand, and life became even more difficult for me. Of course some of the staff joined him because he was a very famous and extremely popular hairdresser for so many years. This was the time I had no choice but to bring Sacha from Essensuals to help me run Toni & Guy full-time. I felt I was very quickly up against it and really it was the only way to survive. If I hadn't had Sacha to call on, I think we really would have gone under. I desperately needed help and I am so grateful I had Sacha to turn to – it's the truth. At that point I felt I was fighting for my life, and the only way I know is to work harder and harder.

I went into Toni & Guy accessories to try to get some distributors in there. It was hard to get some people to come to our school and with all honesty I think it was touch and go before it worked. It was the start of my recovery, but it still wasn't making enough money so we concentrated on consolidating existing business and developing more Toni & Guy salons, in the UK and overseas. My overtures were not always successful It was a very challenging situation and for a time it was extremely difficult and stressful. But after a while I found that I had started to enjoy myself again. It was a wonderful feeling – taking on a big challenge is a good way of life. I was free from the influence of my brothers too. As time went on and the business improved, thanks so much to Sacha's efforts, I felt like a bird set free to fly wherever it wants to go. I never dreamt it would rise to be so successful. In those difficult days after the demerger I had no great expectations. *If I end up with just a few salons, so be it*, I thought.

I had no fear and little by little, I started doing more and more expansions. The pace was frenetic. In 2003 we opened Toni & Guy salons around Britain – in Grimsby, Basingstoke, Bath, Belfast, Braintree, Crewe, Epping, Lakeside, Market Harborough, Marlow, Swansea, Walsall and Wigan; and in London – in Clapham Junction, Liverpool Street, Paddington Central and Victoria. Abroad, we opened salons in Dubai, Thailand, Portugal, Italy, Cyprus and two new salons in both Germany and Australia. In 2004 we opened Toni & Guy salons in Andover, Dorchester, Fleet, Kendal, Leatherhead, Liverpool, Newark, Oldham, Oswestry, Redditch, Stockton Heath, Teddington and Telford; and in London in Crouch End, Fenchurch Street and Great Portland Street. Abroad, we opened Toni & Guy salons in Ireland, Indonesia, France and Cyprus, and two new salons in Italy, two in Greece and nine in Australia. And we maintained the momentum. We opened fourteen more British salons in 2005, and twenty-one abroad in countries from Russia to Japan and from Norway to China. It swiftly became an exciting, exhilarating time.

Of course it was not just a matter of opening new salons, important though that most certainly was. At the same time I tried very hard to find top-quality new and different products to market. I widened the range and developed more Toni & Guy products, always trying to make the very best I could. We had a lot of positive publicity, thanks partly to the huge growth in America, which everybody still identified as just part of one family business. They still saw me as being the head of the family, which was obviously a point of view I did not discourage. In my heart many times I genuinely felt that we were still a family business together; blood is stronger than anything else. I announced nothing about the difficult details of the division and just said that the two parts of the business had each taken a different direction, which was the truth. We were still a very close family, and we still are today.

Life was more argumentative before but Italians are passionate people: we still argue, but not about business. And we still tried to see each other whenever we could, as we still do. I visit my brothers in the US and they come over to England for family reunions and occasions. It is wonderful that all the children get on very well together. Nothing was done in a bad manner. In a way we just had our differences and then settled them so we had no choice but to move on. I would love to have had one company globally, but that was no longer possible so Sacha and I felt that we had to concentrate on running the Toni & Guy we were left with as well and as profitably as possible.

It was a very intensive period of work. I did a lot of newspaper and magazine interviews and consequently there was a great deal of good publicity. I also spent a lot of time with the American comedienne and presenter Ruby Wax, who was making a television programme about Toni & Guy. She was determined to 'dish the dirt' and tried hard to discover if my brothers and I had split after a huge acrimonious row. But of course that was ridiculous so she never managed to produce any juicy revelations at all. She was disappointed but she should not have blamed herself because there had been no bust-up and the business gradually improved and developed all over again. I had a high profile, and I used it. I'd been helped because in 2000 I had been named London Entrepreneur of the Year in the Consumer Products and Services category of the London Entrepreneur of the Year Awards and Toni & Guy started winning more Hairdresser of the Year Awards.

I was very flattered by the Entrepreneur Award but in all honesty I feel, in my case particularly, it was more about desperately wanting to fulfil a need than any great gift. I believe anyone can be an entrepreneur if there is a need either for them or for their family or the market. That's how you become an entrepreneur. You can't just wake up and be an entrepreneur, you have to need it; I needed franchises. When you need something, you invent it so I adapted franchises to fit hairdressing salons and made them profitable. It was the same earlier when I needed money for my children's education: I invented a way to pay the school fees. When I needed funds to grow my business, I started my own personal pension trust – it became my own bank.

In all honesty I do not believe there is really such a thing as an entrepreneur. There are just people who rise to the occasion and fulfil a need, either for themselves or for their family, or if they really need to get something done for whatever reason. I needed to grow the business and safeguard my family. I believe that in life and in business the more you give, the more you get back. And, of course, the less you give, the less you get back. I think that is really true. My philosophy is never to make anyone redundant and to treat everybody as a member of one great big happy family. As I've said before, it's 'All for one, one for all' in my business. If I need to safeguard my team I will take reduced wages myself and in some cases no wages at all. In that worst case I would think, *So be it*, for that is my job at the end of the day.

★　★　★

If you enjoy your job, and you should because you spend most of your life working at it, then you are not doing it purely for the money. So if you begin to make extra money, why not spend it on your salons to make them more comfortable for yourself and your clients? I believe you shouldn't think about the money when you are doing the job. If you do it to the best of your ability, the money will come automatically. Hairdressers should always remember that the clients don't just want their hair done, they also want a consultation and a pleasant experience. They want to know about style and fashion and all the latest exciting developments and that's why we sponsor London Fashion Week.

In the past we had established this enormous reputation for our artistic style, which was second to none. We had won lots of awards and the education was very powerful and important for us. When we were left in charge after the demerger my daughter and I had our very clear tasks to take on. I had to go on and open more and more salons and look after the business side, while Sacha worked hard to improve our image and the education. She exceeded my wildest expectations – and her own, I am sure – for she achieved far more than I could ever have imagined. With her fashion and image knowledge and influence she excelled. She is such an intelligent and elegant woman too and also a great leader. Her husband, James Tarbuck, was very supportive and with Sacha moving to Toni & Guy, her brother Christian then took control of Essensuals. It was a chance for him to grab hold of with both hands and that's exactly what he did, which made me very happy. He soon started learning about business and he has made tremendous progress. Today he is a very strong businessman. Although I still feel he is an extremely talented hairdresser, he is a great educator, and as an educator he has acquired some of our top franchisees and taught them himself. Christian is a very gifted young man and I think the time will come when he will shine through even more.

There is no alternative to hard work and after the demerger I worked harder than ever, undertaking a world tour in 2002. This time I decided to take Christian with me and we went on a worldwide trip around some of our furthest-flung outposts. I was anxious to consolidate and to reassure as many of our key franchisees as possible that it was business as usual, only more so. We travelled first to the opening of Toni & Guy Bangkok. The reaction from the people of Thailand was warm and welcoming and their cheerful enthusiasm helped recharge my batteries. Local press and TV coverage was very encouraging and we developed plans to create a chain of both Toni & Guy salons and Essensuals throughout the country.

From Thailand we flew to Hong Kong, where we visited the staff of the newly opened Toni & Guy salon, which was very impressive. Then we flew on to New Zealand, where we discussed some exciting plans to open a string of Toni & Guy salons across that beautiful country.

The next stop was Australia, where I visited both Sydney and Melbourne. Australia had become a highly successful platform for Toni & Guy, with steady growth and strong education and marketing. With one of my top executives, Dennis Langford, I drew up projections for major growth for the next few years for both Toni & Guy and Essensuals. Even then I didn't stop. Barely had my feet touched English soil (there was just a brief break at home) than I was off again, this time to Russia, for the opening of Toni & Guy Moscow. Shaun Hunt, who had previously worked in Knightsbridge, had been working with the Russian team for a couple of months and together they put on a fabulous fashion show on a specially created catwalk in the square outside the salon. There was a fantastic party with Anastasia Volochkova, the principal ballerina with the Bolshoi Ballet, as our special guest. But my travels were still not over and so I visited Italy and the Toni & Guy salons in Como, Florence and Verona.

In 2003 we founded the Toni & Guy Charitable Foundation, a fund-raising organisation with the initial aim of opening a new children's ward at King's College Hospital in London for young patients with liver and heart problems. The target was £700,000 but we raised well over half in the first three years.

We also built a hostel and forty-eight apartments in Italy, working closely with the local priest. The apartments are to help house a variety of desolate lost young souls. I was always brought up to show charity to people. As a boy I would give up my seat on the bus to an adult and I would often help an old lady across the road. But later, when I had a young family of my own in London, I worked eighteen hours a day seven days a week to put a roof over their heads and give them an education so there was no time for charity. Once they were all grown up and our business had prospered there was time and I wanted to use it to help other people. My first major charity was the hostel and apartments, Fondazione Oasi Regina degli Angeli in Ameglio in southern Italy, which offers shelter for children who are disadvantaged due to physical or psychological problems. In the UK we started by supporting the Variety Club, but when my wife and I visited King's College Hospital and saw how many children's lives could be saved for the cost of opening four or five salons, we set up the Toni & Guy Charitable Foundation to sponsor a ward.

Sometimes it is more important to give time than money. In business I might let someone off a month's bills, but it is usually better if I speak to them and try to motivate them. It's the same with charity, although of course money is also very important. The Toni & Guy Foundation employs only one salaried person to co-ordinate donations and spending. All other work is done on a voluntary basis and we use the Toni & Guy offices for free so more than 95 per cent of the money that comes in goes directly to the hospital.

I think it is important that the ward we sponsor is known as the Toni & Guy Ward so that people know who donated the funds. It is important because of pride and because we have 5,000 hairdressers who'll be more inclined to support something we've done ourselves. We don't just give because we want people to know we are generous, and sometimes I give secretly but when it comes to the hospital ward I think promoting the company is a good thing.

I know that I'm fortunate to be in a position to be able to help others but I think we should all try to help those in need. When I see people in the street I am torn. I remember once walking past a young girl who was begging and it bothered me so much that a few minutes later, I got so upset that I ran back to give her something. But although I looked everywhere, I couldn't find her. However, I do believe that sometimes we should put our own country first. Indeed it was Mother Teresa of Calcutta who once told my wife that everyone was helping children in India and Africa and not worrying enough about the unfortunates in their own countries.

Over the years I'm delighted to say that our efforts for charity have expanded enormously. We have developed a partnership with Macmillan Cancer Support and also worked extensively with The

Prince's Trust, the Stroke Association and Crimestoppers. To date we have raised more than £1.5 million for good causes. I'm very proud of our record and I pledge that we will go on to raise much more of the money that is so badly needed.

Sacha helped me to see the remarkable potential of developing the sale of products. She agreed with me that everything has to be first class when it comes to quality. My whole life has been about the pursuit of excellence. When we introduced our new product range, label.m, in 2004 it was all brilliantly created and overseen by Sacha with exactly the same driving principle of always striving to be the best. With label.m, we tried from the start to make the most stylish and attractive products possible. We didn't care how much they cost, and this in turn helped to make us successful. The thinking behind it was *The young people will be the ones who are the strength of the company*.

You've got to trust, and I trust everybody at Toni & Guy. My artistic team is absolutely brilliant; there is no better team anywhere. But I trust myself even more, because I have known what to do with a pair of hairdressing scissors since I was twelve years old.

I always monitor the structure of the salon so that I can be ready to make any changes we might need. Nothing ever stays the same, things are always changing – it is very important to accept that. The entrance has to be smart and clean and then you need a beautiful changing room and toilets, you also need comfortable basins where you can relax and feel refreshed. You need light and images all around you. When clients think about Toni & Guy their expectations are very high – so you have got to be prepared because everything must be geared towards giving them the best. Fundamentally, you have to have huge respect for your customers. That is the Toni & Guy message and I hope it always will be.

Courage is also very important. I often tell the story of a guy I once knew who had a fantastic salon, great looks, great training and everything going for him, but he did not make it because he lacked one crucial thing: courage. As well as everything else I have talked about, you need courage and determination to go on and make your dream come true.

Label.m was fully launched internationally in 2006 and it gave the company a huge instant boost. The new products were an immediate hit and Toni & Guy just became stronger and stronger. We became the first hairdressing salon ever to be voted a Superbrand, which was the amazing accolade we won in 2005 and 2006. Then we became a CoolBrand, which was fantastic. I was extremely proud and of course pleased for all our employees. It was a good time in my life, but then I am fortunate enough to have had many good times. We had almost 5,000 employees in Britain and another 3,500 across the world. The annual turnover had reached £175 million. a remarkable eleven times and pioneered extras to the salon service such as videos, a magazine and even our own dedicated TV station.

Of course as the business grew so too did the challenges it represented. I was always determined to keep the same highest standards of service across all the salons, wherever they were. And I've never altered from wanting to encourage creativity and maintain the family atmosphere so vital to our ongoing success. We have salons from China to Australia. The people who run them are all ex-employees, there is not one person who did not start out by working with us. Our first franchisee in Japan (Kenjo Saiga) had started out with us in 1973! His two boys came to work for me in London. The older one took over the franchise from his father. That's the kind of family continuity I love, and it is one of the great benefits of being in it for the long haul. There was also a German franchisee whose son now works for us. If anyone wants to open a Toni & Guy franchise they have to work with the company for something like six, seven or eight years at least first. It is very much an internal family thing – Toni & Guy is a business that builds from within.

Long ago I realised that life does not stay the same. As times and fashions move on, it is extremely important to keep changing along with the market. Sacha's youthful energy and drive helped us more than I can say. Together we strengthened the brand considerably and label.m has become a product that has grown unbelievably – it's really the best brand in the market place. We have enjoyed huge success, particularly in the United States with organic products, and now we are established and growing all over the world.

In October 2006 I received a very great honour from the country of my birth. The Cavaliere Ufficiale is the Italian equivalent of the British knighthood. Its full title is Cavaliere Ufficiale dell'Ordine al Merito della Repubblica Italiana and it was bestowed on me in a very emotional ceremony at the Italian Embassy in London for my 'Contribution to Italian business'. I was so pleased Pauline, Sacha, Christian and Pierre were all with me. It was a very moving occasion. I made a speech, which went down well, but afterwards I couldn't remember a single word of what I had said! I felt very honoured but also a little embarrassed because I hadn't done anything in Italy. I've done everything for Britain. But there you are, that's how it goes. I was very, very honoured and would never have wanted anything else. As well as my family to witness my big moment I had with me a bishop, nine priests and around 140 friends, relatives and business acquaintances. It was wonderful!

Then two years later I was so happy to be awarded an honorary

British OBE. 'In recognition of his services to British hairdressing, Giuseppe Toni Mascolo was presented with an honorary OBE,' said the official announcement. I was extremely moved and grateful, not just for myself but for my family and everyone who has worked for Toni & Guy. It was presented to me by the then Secretary of State for Culture, Media and Sport, Andy Burnham. A traditionalist at heart, I believe it came direct from HM the Queen. I was thrilled to be given this honour by Her Majesty. To receive an OBE was wonderful. Starting from a small shop in south London and then moving the business on to a worldwide stage was a lifetime's work I undertook for my family. I said how exciting it was to head a company that inspires hairdressers and pointed out that our London Academy attracted thousands of overseas visitors and this, coupled with the global export of our hairdressing education and haircare ranges, had helped us to play a vital part in Britain's outstanding contribution to the world of hairdressing.

Of course I would have preferred to receive the honour from Her Majesty but Andy Burnham was very gracious. And he had done his homework. He said: 'In the world of hairdressing the Toni & Guy brand is synonymous with cutting-edge style, progressive creativity and inspiration. Toni's emphasis on training and education has helped Britain's hairdressing industry become a global leader in the cutting and styling of hair, showing the world the kind of creativity this country can produce.'

I was thrilled to receive the OBE and it was great because everyone in my family was happy. I know my life can look as if it is one big happy success story, but of course that is not the case. Over the years I have made many mistakes but I think I have learned something from every one of them. And I try not to make big mistakes. I never bear grudges – I don't like it if someone lets me down but where possible, I believe in giving people a second chance.

In 2007 I stepped in to rescue our main franchisee in Ireland after his operation hit difficulties and came close to bankruptcy. We sent in our people to sort it out. He had made a mistake but he went back to the salons and was working hard.

The business is such an important part of my life. For me family, business and pleasure are all wound up together. I think one of my strengths is that I am flexible, especially in franchising. Pretty well every deal is negotiated on an individual basis. Some people seem surprised at that but every person is different and every salon is different even if I do always demand the same high standards. I like to handle as many deals as possible personally. Everyone has my mobile number and sometimes I have to be dragged away when I start chatting to employees. I love people and I love the hairdressing business. Always I come back to one of our mottoes: 'Education, teamwork, communication and motivation' – that's what it's all about. Some people ask if I have ever been to business school. I haven't, but I have sent others.

I've seen countless famous faces come through the doors of my salons over the year – people like Gregory Peck, Diana Ross and some of the Rolling Stones, to name but a few. I've even cut Dame Edna's hair as Barry Humphries is a regular customer. But I don't think I've ever influenced an election before Boris Johnson came in for a haircut the night before the vote for mayor of London in 2008. He had all that wild and bushy hair when he came in, but after we gave him a great haircut, he was suddenly presentable. And he won, didn't he? I like to think the haircut helped!

Of course Boris is a colourful character but I very much enjoy meeting people from all walks of life. Richard Branson has been perhaps my greatest influence. He's done difficult things and made a success; he's also very courageous, strong and not afraid of anybody. As an entrepreneur he's second to none. But there are many business people I admire. I think I was in my mid-sixties when people started mentioning the 'R' word, retirement. That's something I was not ready to consider then, and I'm still not. I remember reading that Sir Ken Morrison was making a bid for Safeway when he was seventy-one years old and I was very encouraged. I want to keep going as long as I enjoy it.

I was very happy that Toni & Guy did well and thrived, thanks so much to the great assistance I received from Sacha and James. My brothers Guy, Bruno and Anthony were extremely successful as well, particularly in January 2009 when they sold TIGI to Unilever for some $411 million. Of course it was a great achievement for them but TIGI was a company I created so I felt quite amazed and staggered myself, even though I did not benefit financially. But by then Toni & Guy were doing very, very well, with more than 230 salons in the UK and another 175 worldwide. We were turning over more than £175 million a year so I was happy with how my company was doing.

★ ★ ★

Then, on my birthday in May 2009, came a terrible personal blow. Guy died from a heart attack at his home in Dallas. The news came as a dreadful shock and I was distraught. He was only sixty-five and he had so much to live for. The demerger might have separated the business into two parts but the family remained one – it still does today. Guy and I had always been very close, all our lives. When we started Toni & Guy together we became even closer, I suppose because for a time it was just the two of us, fighting to save the family. We made a great partnership. Guy brought the creativity and artistry, while I had the business sense. He was so handsome and so talented that we were never short of clients. The ladies loved him and so did I. There is not a day that goes by without me thinking about him. I miss him very deeply and I really do believe that Guy was the greatest hairdresser who ever lived.

Whatever happens in life, you have to be constant and keep your mind on the job. It warms my heart when people still say to me: 'I couldn't imagine England without a Toni & Guy.' I was a pioneer, you see, we were the first British brand to bring the franchise model to the UK. The franchise model works particularly well in the hairdressing industry. Once you've trained up a new stylist, the last thing you want is for them to leave and go into competition with you. The answer to that problem is to say: 'Open your own salon. We'll give you the education, the image, the tools, uniforms and so on.' It's much cheaper for them than going it alone, and then we don't lose any of our Toni & Guy family – I'm a bit sentimental about my staff. To date we have trained more than 100,000 hairdressers in twenty-seven Toni & Guy academies worldwide. If they all started up rival businesses, we'd be in big trouble!

We were still expanding in 2009. I opened more salons in France, China, Russia, Australia, and in several Eastern European countries. Russia did extremely well and China was amazing, as I knew it would be. Our label.m boomed brilliantly all over the world. In less than eighteen months we landed fifty distributors in fifty countries. In Australia, we made £750,000 from the range in just three months.

I am always pushing the brand further – you can never underestimate other businesses out there. The moment you come up with something new, everybody jumps on it. Toni & Guy were the first salons to invent the gels and mousses that you see everywhere now. We came up with new methods for cutting and texturising hair. Now everybody does it. It's frustrating! I would be the richest man in England if only I could have trademarked it, but you can't, so I stay alert and compete.

There are many factors in creating a successful business. In a hairdressing salon I have always felt that it begins with reception. An attractive and efficient reception is the heart of your business. It pumps the clients, who are the lifeblood of the enterprise, around the salon without ever missing a beat. The receptionist should be a perfect hostess, focusing entirely on the delight of the customers. Never forget that delighted customers spend more money, have more services and come back more frequently than unhappy ones. The receptionist is as valuable as an amazing stylist or colourist and an essential part of a high-performing team. A really good receptionist can increase the salon takings by at least 20 per cent! Never undervalue your receptionist.

I have always searched for excellence in all employees. The stylists and all team members must of course be first class and the franchisees must be exceptional people – that is part of the Toni & Guy philosophy. I always look first for qualities that come naturally, the ones that are impossible to teach. Number one on my list is passion. It's one of our company values and I believe it is present in all successful people, in those who find their work as fulfilling as a hobby. With passion comes drive and commitment, a fundamental necessity in all departments, and particularly in franchisees. I also look for pride because with pride comes attention to detail and personal standards. Dedication to personal development is also high on my list.

When I look for new franchisees I want to find people who are prepared to give everything in their pursuit of perfection and excellence. I want to find people who are flexible, willing to move with the times and modern in their thinking. All these qualities are essential to help our fast-moving business succeed and stay at number one. We need dedication to learning and improving in order to be the best.

I also look for courage: you need balls to be in business. You need tenacity that will carry you through the tough times as well as the good. There are other necessary qualities but these can be taught and learnt over time. A franchise owner with Toni & Guy must be an amazing and inspirational leader, who is totally in touch with his/her business and at the same time always able to excite, inspire and motivate both clients and team members. When recruiting, we look for caring, creative, curious people, who can foster an environment of trust and respect.

From the start we worked hard to dispel the myth that hairdressers are uneducated with our passion for 'education, education, education'. I always look for people prepared to go the extra mile; those who are prepared to dedicate their own time as well as the company's to perfecting every skill they have. I have long preached that it is no good simply practising your hair skills. It is vital for anyone wishing to succeed in our business to be a master of communication, too, particularly if they want to be a stylist or a technician. All employees are encouraged to learn all they can about the industry they are working in. They should strive to become expert in their skills and to learn every service. I believe they should find a passion for current affairs and for popular culture so that they are able to surprise their clients with the breadth and the depth of their knowledge.

Young people often come in for some harsh criticism from their elders, especially those who are as old as myself. But I do not join in. Because of my own experience I believe I understand their position a little. I know that school-leavers often lack self-confidence. They are unable to use communication to positively influence clients and to manage their relationships with colleagues. And they lack sophistication, tend to bring their problems to work and lack motivation. Their interpersonal skills have not yet been developed because of a lack of experience. They are unable to look a client in the eye and smile and chat. Some lack numeracy, literacy and even IT skills. But I do not know anyone who had such skills when they started off. I can't even think of anyone, even if I think back for fifty years. It's unreasonable to expect too much from school-leavers.

When we take on school-leavers they are not prepared for work and we should not expect them to be. Businesses should drop the unrealistic expectations they sometimes have. We all learned on the job how to deal with a demanding clientele. Interpersonal skills come with patience, good coaching and a fair and realistic time frame. It takes years for doctors and dentists to become expert, during which time they hone their bedside manner as well as fine-tune their practical skills. We hairdressers are no different. I did not leave school with these skills, I learned them by observing older role models. The level we work at now is what has chiefly changed: we have to deliver even more to clients because they have more choice. Today we are far more conscious of the salon experience.

I believe we are failing our youth by not educating them in life skills, especially communication. There are plenty of youngsters who have an amazing approach to life and work; there are those who need more intensive guidance to find their work ethic and then there are those who do not make it, no matter what. If one of our youngsters is failing, I always ask, 'What more could we have done? Why have we not tapped into this youngster's psyche? Why have we not understood how to motivate them?' And you know what, sometimes the answer is, 'We have done all we can,' but sometimes I know we could have done more and that makes me sad.

We deal with it by supporting the youth apprenticeship schemes run by the Government. I heartily support the idea of beginning to educate youngsters in skills for industry from the age of fourteen – I find it exciting to go further than just offering a few weeks' work experience, but to work with youngsters who have chosen hairdressing as their career over a couple of years. We need to have faith and belief in our youth.

I love people and I think that the thing I love most about our industry is how sociable it is. You are daily given the chance to meet and connect with people while learning and developing. I always get more pleasure from giving than receiving and I love it when I know that I have made someone happy. To keep in touch with my craft I still cut hair on Saturdays and I do truly look forward to it but I am fortunate that I thoroughly enjoy just about every aspect of my work. I wish I didn't have to go to sleep at night – I would happily work twenty-four hours a day if my body (and my wife) would allow it!

What helps to keep my life interesting is that Toni & Guy operates in a forever-changing world. I love that and it makes my blood boil when I find people, particularly employees, who are reluctant to move with the times, who live in the past and are unable to move on. When I go into London each Saturday to run a column of clients it's the highlight of my week. I look forward to seeing my clients. Some of them I have grown up with and I've watched their careers flourish but others are new friends with new ideas and demands, and they help to keep me on my toes. I like to try all the new products and equipment and the new toys I can show off to the clients. It's wonderful to get paid when you are having such a great time! The biggest reward in my job though is making people look and feel great. Sometimes people ask me about retirement but I never give it a thought.

People often ask me for the secret of my success. I always try to answer honestly and my answer is, obviously, the ability to work very hard and to always have the aim of developing things and always doing the best job you can for your clients. It's not about the money. More important than anything else I always say to all my staff, 'If you think all the time about making money then you are never going to make money because obviously your mind will not be on your job. If you think about giving the best service and treating the client like a guest, and doing the best you can, then you might make more money.'

I have always wanted clients to be welcomed as if they were coming to your house. In that case you would do the best to entertain them with courtesy and good food – and possibly a great glass of wine. You just do your best to make guests welcome if they come into your home and I believe it should be exactly the same with the clients who come into your salon. I remember from the early days if a new client came to Sloane Square, I would show them the upstairs and the downstairs of our very elegant salon. For me it was like someone coming to visit my family – I always knew that it was most important that they should feel part of the family when they came in.

Right from the start I had that attitude. I remember clients coming in and saying: 'It's amazing here, so welcoming and so relaxed.' And then they would sometimes add: 'You look really tired and busy. Can I go and make you a cup of tea?' So that was customer service in reverse! We started in Clapham with precisely the same philosophy that drives on Toni & Guy now: we helped each other, we worked for each other, we shared ideas and we communicated with each other. Although fifty years have gone by, that philosophy has not changed.

I said: 'Education, education, education' long before Tony Blair did, but when he was beginning his challenge to become Prime Minister, I saw him at the Albert Hall and I said then: 'Look, this young man is going to have a landslide and become the next Prime Minister because he believes in "education, education, education".' I always knew it was a winning formula – I had that in my mind even in the Clapham days, even though it was then a totally new concept. We had to create something new out of learning and dedication to our business. Everything I have done since then has all been linked to the same philosophy.

The year 2013 was very special as it marked our fiftieth anniversary. Who could have imagined a little hairdressing salon in Clapham set up in 1963 would lead to a chain of salons spanning the world? In 2013 I set out to visit as many of our salons and talk to as many of our employees as I possibly could. It was exhausting but I had some wonderful trips. I went to South Korea and to China, where we did a show in the open in the middle of Beijing, then to Russia, where I was heartened to see how much everyone wanted to meet me! In Moscow we did a wonderful show in the street and then we went on to do shows in Singapore, Australia and Italy.

As always it was fantastic to see the worldwide success of Toni & Guy. So how do I feel now? I feel so moved by the business that

I started so long ago and have guided through the years. I used to think that without me it could collapse but now I know that I've got a great team that I trust to carry on, way into the future. Not that I'm considering retiring! Today I'm feeling like the same kid I was when I started it all. I feel the same energy and drive and I want to go on forever.

Some things will never change — I treat everybody the same, I don't treat anybody differently. I don't like those toffee-nosed people who look down on others. I am proud and content, but I know you are just as good as your last haircut. No one can rest on his laurels, and I certainly never will. I am going forward all the time, there is always a new thing, because that is what my life is: a journey. I may never arrive, but always I am on a journey to achieving as much as I can. And I will work, work, work, till I die. My family is my enjoyment. My enjoyment is not going to the pub and having beers, but working all the time so my family will always be happy and safe.

I never cease to be surprised and amazed by the turns my life takes and so I was deeply moved when Pauline and I were honoured with the award of a Papal Knighthood in March 2013. The Catholic Church paid this enormous tribute, which was bestowed personally by Pope Benedict XVI. In fact it was one of his last acts before his retirement. Pauline and I became a Knight and a Dame Commander of Saint Gregory in a deeply moving ceremony in Southwark Cathedral of all places — where we were married. The honour was presented by Archbishop Peter Smith at a special private mass with our family, friends and colleagues in the congregation. Afterwards we had a beautiful champagne reception and dinner at the Ritz. It was a wonderful day that neither Pauline nor I will ever forget.

The most amazing awards seem to keep coming. I was very moved recently to be made an honorary professor at Durham University Business School. And the Fellowship of British Hairdressers gave me a 'Lifetime Achievement Award'. I am only the second person to receive such an accolade. The only other person to receive one was Vidal Sassoon. It was awarded just a few days before he died in 2012. At the ceremony I joked: 'Look, I don't want it: I'm not ready to go yet!'

My focus has always been strengthening the company, improving the product and helping the franchises to expand more and more – Kazakhstan, Saudi Arabia, Indonesia, China, India, Argentina, and then, who knows?

I know we have achieved a great deal with Toni & Guy but deep down in my heart, in all honesty I truly feel that *We've only just begun…*

CHAPTER TWENTY-ONE

A SPECIAL FAMILY: THE FIFTIETH ANNIVERSARY

Sunday, 8 September 2013 is a day that was in my diary for a long time, but will live in my heart for even longer. The Fiftieth Anniversary Festival of Toni & Guy was a day of celebration that I will never, ever forget. It was another wonderful date in the amazing calendar of our extraordinary family business. The Festival was a fabulous occasion that far surpassed my wildest aspirations and became one of the most unforgettable days of my life.

In the beautiful grounds of historic Knebworth House, which have been graced over the years by a long list of famous international figures, from Sir Winston Churchill and Mick Jagger to Her Majesty the Queen and Charles Dickens, more than 5,000 members of our far-flung Toni & Guy family came together to celebrate our extraordinary landmark birthday party. I don't believe any other hairdressing company has staged a music festival to mark their fiftieth anniversary. The idea for the tremendous coming together came, not surprisingly, from my daughter Sacha, who specialises in original thinking to the extreme!

I found it almost overwhelming to see so many of my Toni & Guy people in one place at the same time. Today we have more than 400 salons in no fewer than forty-one different countries and we have more than 8,000 employees all over the world. I was delighted to see so many of them had made the journey to be with us for our truly fabulous Festival. They came from the furthest corners of the globe, from Australia and China, from Switzerland and Saudi Arabia. To me it was quite staggering and deeply moving to see them all converge on this beautiful corner of Hertfordshire with exactly the same idea in mind: they all wanted to have a great big family party to say happy fiftieth birthday to Toni & Guy. I was just so delighted to see them all. Everywhere I looked there were smiles and you could hear whoops of laughter as old friends from far and wide met and enjoyed each other's company all over again.

It was a real joy for me to see our huge Toni & Guy family congregating in such beautiful surroundings and enjoying themselves. Every minute of the day was a pleasure filled with so many highs, but most of all I think my favourite moments were spent meeting old friends from long past. So many Toni & Guy people have worked with us for decades. I believe it is a tribute to our family business that we have so many members who have been with us for very many years. As my family have said, I always hate it when anyone leaves Toni & Guy because to me they are genuinely part of my family. The great thing is that departures from our company do not happen very often. We have a large number of very long-serving employees, which I believe speaks volumes about the sort of company we are. Our people are our family and our strength. I always try to meet and talk to as many of our people as often as I can, but of course under normal circumstances I am limited by the fact that they are spread all over the world. That afternoon gave me a wonderful chance to meet so many friends, old and new.

The Festival was all brilliantly organised by my daughter Sacha with her sensational sense of flair and imagination. It ran from 2 pm until 2 am and there was something for everyone, from fairground rides to a fashion show and from a great parkland party to a magical musical concert. Even the weather co-operated. Early in the afternoon the heavens did dare to open for a mercifully short time and we all enjoyed a little September shower. Thanks to Sacha's foresight, Toni & Guy umbrellas were swiftly available for all – she really does seem to think of everything. But after the unscheduled downpour the day really brightened up in every way. I really enjoyed walking around and meeting the many, many people who came to celebrate half a century of hairdressing success with us.

The music began early in the afternoon on the outdoor second stage and it certainly lifted the spirits of all concerned. There were stylish stalls serving quality food and drinks, and the rides were swiftly in full swing. After taking a careful look I decided against going on the 'Extreme' fairground ride which whirled people high in the air, way above the party. Someone has to keep his feet on the ground!

Backstage, the preparations began even earlier in the day because some of the styles to be seen on the catwalk in the main stage extravaganza later were enormously elaborate and took hours to create. Because we were celebrating fifty years of Toni & Guy there were lots of echoes of previous popular styles. I was particularly delighted to see a variation on the theme of Anthony's famous

'Veil' hairstyle, which was so inspirational and important to us. Yet it was certainly not the only style that brought back happy memories.

The afternoon was a great time for meeting old friends, and not all of them were from the world of hairdressing. For example, Mr Andrew Love is the deputy chairman of the famous Ritz hotel in London and I got to know him through working to help raise money for the Stroke Association. But I will let him explain:

I've never been to anything like Toni & Guy's 50th Anniversary Festival. It was an entertaining and eye-opening experience; I wouldn't have missed it for the world. I don't know much about hairdressing but I know happy employees when I see them and Knebworth had thousands on show that afternoon.

I got to know Toni Mascolo because we both suffered strokes and were fortunate enough to make a full recovery. We then became involved in fund-raising for the main stroke charity. I guess that brought us together in more ways than one. Toni is a remarkable chap – he is very polite, quiet and mild-mannered but hugely energetic, successful and extremely generous. Lots of people talk a lot about raising money and doing good. Toni says very little and contributes greatly, both with his time as well as with money; he's a great guy. He does a lot of generous things that very few people know about. And he certainly knows how to throw a party!

The Festival felt absolutely fantastic to me but I would like to let some of the franchisees and employees who travelled from all over the world to be with us explain how the day felt to them. Of course not everyone came a long way. Franchisee Carl McCaffrey had one of the shortest journeys from our Canary Wharf salon in London, but his is one of our most successful businesses. I wanted to hear from him.

Carl said:

Toni & Guy is the top hairdressing business in the world and I've got their number one salon in the world for turnover. Canary Wharf is a diamond and I love polishing it.

I believe that one of Toni's great strengths is the way that he trusts you and leaves you alone to run the business. He doesn't interfere and in the whole scheme of business and competition he is a complete gentleman. But if you ever need any help or advice he is there for you. I definitely do not mean that he is soft. If you do something he does not like or approve of then you very quickly find out.

If you're on the 'naughty step', Toni is very clear: you're told you're on the 'naughty step' and you very quickly mend your ways. He is very straight. Now he's got 240 salons in the UK and he makes them survive because he is very dedicated and he knows his business. In recent years Toni & Guy have taken some salons back because a lot of the franchisees were not performing, presumably because they had lost their libido or appetite. It's sad, but it happens. I am forty years old now and I've been with Toni for twenty years. I am especially fortunate because I have been allowed to open a second salon, a brand-new one. So I've got a wonderful new place to work, with a wonderful brand. I'm a happy man, I've got forty-five staff and it's a good unit. In fact, it's a machine that's very nicely oiled, and doing very well indeed.

Toni is so kind and gentle. He has great strength of character, but he is always very calm and measured. If there is a problem or a disagreement, he doesn't get angry, he just gets on with it. He is one of those guys who is just naturally devoted to the job and to his family. He has been through a lot, with his health problems and with the loss of his brother, and I know sometimes in business you have to wonder who's your enemy and who's your friend. I've been with the brand for twenty years and it's genuinely like being in a family. My best friend is Sacha and I can never see myself working anywhere else. I think I am very lucky, but then again, they're very lucky to have me!

I was a bit painful four years ago – I could have been sacked, back then, for my behaviour. I think I was playing around a bit and behaving as if I was a rock star and probably not being discreet. You have got to appreciate what you have, but the thing is I've known Toni for twenty years and I'm very lucky that they brought me in and said, 'You've been a naughty boy. You either get your act together or you lose it.' It was a turning point for me and it was when I realised how lucky I was to have someone who cared about me and loved me. Working for Toni & Guy has been fabulous – it's a great big happy family that I never want to leave!

As I walked around the Festival I met so many people who have worked with us for years. I was pleased to see so many had made the trip and some had travelled from all over the world. Sean Rowse has the franchises in Switzerland and I'll let him explain what Toni & Guy means to him.

Sean said:

I've got the franchises in Switzerland, in Geneva, Zurich, Basle and Lugano, and I can't speak highly enough of working with Toni & Guy. I was working in Bath and I'd spent a couple of years working for Toni & Guy and I wanted to try to get my own franchise. I decided the Channel Islands would be a great place to start, so I went out and found premises there and it all started for me. That was the first time I had ever met Toni. It was a very big organisation and at first that enormous size was quite frightening and intimidating for me. I had worked for the company for two years and Toni had become such a huge icon in the fashion business. I remember I was very nervous about meeting him face to face, but in the end when I finally did come face to face with him he was so relaxed and friendly, it was a real pleasure.

He came over with his wife Pauline to Jersey and we went to look at shops. We found a good place and we opened a salon there. After that I got to know him better and liked working with him very much. He was fantastic again when I wanted to start to develop more salons. My career with Toni & Guy is great and so much of that is down to the man at the top. I will always be grateful to him because I know that I owe him a very great deal.

After being very apprehensive before we met I was delighted when my first impression of Toni was such a massive relief: he was just very open and straight. We sat and talked and he showed me plans for new salons and other products. He is a remarkable individual, so normal and so down to earth. He is very successful and has achieved so much, it would be understandable if he was full of himself but I was very pleased to discover there were no airs and graces about Toni

Mascolo. He just talked really naturally to me and he was really interesting and ever since then whenever I see him since he always remembers everything.

It was not easy to switch over to running salons in Switzerland. It was difficult to build up the four salons because although obviously you know the platform in the UK, you have to try to establish that in Switzerland, which is a very different country. We opened Geneva, the first salon in Switzerland, four and a half years ago and what we had to do first was to understand the Swiss laws. Everything about our business was in English and we had to take that into a new country and translate and understand all the laws about shops and rentals and businesses. But Switzerland is such an international place, where there are a many American and British people, which made it a lot easier as they and the other international clients were familiar with Toni & Guy. They came into the salons and spread the word a little, which made it easier.

The different languages make it more difficult, because in Geneva it's French, in Zurich it's German, and then you've got Lugano, which is Italian. Those aspects of having to translate everything do still cause problems sometimes. Of course Toni is very understanding and helpful, and thanks to his assistance the salons are proving to be successful, but it is a hard road. We are gradually establishing a platform to show Switzerland what Toni & Guy stands for, and trying to build on that. I believe in the future we could possibly have another eight or nine Toni & Guy salons.

I don't believe this would have been possible without a boss like Toni – he is a great guy. Like many of his people I have been to his house and enjoyed a wonderful time there. Toni

& Guy really is a great big family. Look at the people here at the Festival – there are smiles everywhere you look. Most people stay with Toni & Guy for a long time. I started off as an assistant twenty-odd years ago and now I'm a franchise owner, which is great. It is fantastic to be able to develop your career with one good firm; it gives you a great sense of belonging and security. You can do your own thing, but you always have that brand behind you. You can go to Toni with anything and he will support you and find help for you, and that is the biggest bonus of being in this business. When you open a new salon, wherever it is, you need all the help you can get. You have to learn that quickly and try to get help from other people, and Toni is great at that. He was fantastic when I was first starting, to give me help and support. He always says he is on the end of a telephone and he always has been whenever I've needed help and advice. I'll always be grateful to him.

You might think that in a huge company you would have to go through loads of layers of executives to get to the top, but you don't have that with Toni & Guy. I can just phone Toni up if I've got a problem and ask his advice, and I have done that a few times. He has certainly been very influential in who I am and who I want to be.

One of our very first franchisees was Darren Brewster. He runs our Brighton salon extremely well, and has done so for many years and is one of the senior members of the Toni & Guy family. Darren has a very positive story of years of success with us, but I'll let him explain.

Darren says:

I joined Toni & Guy when I was nineteen and working for them and with them has been a joy – I feel very fortunate. Guy was a brilliant hairdresser and Toni was a fantastic businessman. Anthony came along and was a fabulous flamboyant hairdresser, while Bruno was more like Toni. Together, the brothers were just amazing, there was never a dull moment! They were all motivated and powered by their love of hairdressing much more than for the love of making money and I respect them so much for that.

I started on 11 September 1988 and it is a date I will never forget. I am so lucky to have joined Toni & Guy. This 50th Festival is simply wonderful – there are so many friends sharing so many marvellous memories, I don't want the day to end. Toni has always been a terrific support to me. When we were setting up in Brighton, both Toni and Pauline came down to take a look at the new shop.

Toni was so helpful and accessible then and the most remarkable thing to me is that he still is! You can ring him up at any time and you can always get through to him in person. I can't imagine another top businessman who is so in touch with his people – there is not another hairdressing business like it. In fact, I don't really believe there is another business like it at all!

Like Carl and Sean, Darren is very kind with his comments and like so many of our people he has become a good friend and an important part of our family.

As I wandered around the Festival, happy to meet all these bright young people so clearly having a good time, I felt very proud. Who on earth would have thought that two young Italian brothers who set off in business in the most difficult of circumstances in a humble hairdressing salon in south London would create a huge and successful business empire spanning the globe, half a century later? Not me, for one.

Ever since my brother Guy and I first opened the doors of our little Clapham salon it had been my dream and my driving ambition to build and develop Toni & Guy into my ideal family company. That dream has come true for me and my family and I thank God for our good fortune. But Guy's tragic death in 2009 has been a sorrow in my heart: and on this wonderful day for our business, of all people, Guy should have been with me. I can't help but feel Toni & Guy is always a little incomplete without Guy so I was very happy that his widow, Flora, came to the Festival.

Flora said:

This is a wonderful occasion and I am very glad to be here. I knew Guy Mascolo for twenty-seven years and twenty-seven hours and I still miss him every day.

My personal story is from rags to riches. I was the nanny when I met Guy and we fell in love and eventually married. It was amazing to join such a huge and happy family. Little did I know what I was entering! I was Guy's nanny for his son Zak. I fell head over heels in love with Guy but I had not a clue of what I was really about to take on. I am delighted – you don't know how proud I feel today.

Toni really embraced me as a new member of the family. I felt like one of his daughters, so to speak. He really was kind to me. He and Guy were very close, but very different. Guy was very outgoing and relaxed; Toni was really kind and he always had his own space. He was a little bit sad and serious, but really loving. He was brilliant with the business and a family man at the end. Guy was an ambassador and a peacemaker for the family. I believe the tragedy of their mother's early death had a great impact on both Toni and Guy.

I think that terrible loss was what drove them on and really brought the family unit together; I have no doubt about that. Everybody really strove for the common good. As I look around me now I have to remember the core of what we are. We are family, and we always will be. The Festival is a wonderful way of celebrating that.

As the sun went down on all the outdoor socialising everyone converged on the huge marquee, which was the setting for Sacha's sensational show. The music from the second stage was replaced by entertainment inside a huge and packed arena where the atmosphere, I was delighted to see, was like a giant family party. The audience seemed in extremely high spirits – I don't think I've ever seen so many happy people in one place before. I was absolutely delighted by the response, even when my own speech of welcome was partially drowned out by shouting and applause. I think most people heard me trying to say how proud and happy I was to be celebrating fifty years of Toni & Guy.

I have to admit all the noise of the cheering took me by surprise. What I was trying to say was simply: 'Thank you all for coming, I am really so proud to participate in fifty years of Toni & Guy. I'm so happy to be here, I get so much strength from you. That's what helps me to work with Toni & Guy all these years. I must thank Sacha and Christian and Pierre and James, and everyone. Without you, Toni & Guy couldn't have been the brand that it is today. Thank you for giving us so much help, thank you for helping us to celebrate this wonderful event, thank you to all the guests who have come. I know you have all played a part in our story.'

Sacha masterminded the whole event quite brilliantly. Again, I would like her to speak for herself about a task that added so much to her already-heavy workload.

Sacha says:

I am just so happy that it made my dad happy – that is all that really mattered to me. The Festival did take a lot of planning and preparation but it became so important to me, I did not mind all the extra hours it took. My husband, James, was a great help throughout, as he always is. We have done many, many shows over the years but this one just had to be bigger and better.

I was just so happy when everyone reacted so wonderfully to my dad. When he started to speak there was a huge spontaneous cheer and it almost drowned what he was trying to say, but it really gave me a lift. I've worked really hard, organising the Festival, and it was all for my dad. He deserved a great show and I was determined to give him one. He is such a special person that I had to deliver a special show.

I think it was more than just special: to me it was extra special. I loved every single moment of it. We gave out all the awards for the top salons and our top performers and then put on such a fabulous show of fashion and fantastic hairstyles. I am always amazed to see what our brilliant creative people can come up with and this year it was extra special. With sixty models in action and some quick-change excellence behind the scenes, it seemed as though amazing styles were served up non-stop. It was very impressive. Sacha made sure we showcased Toni & Guy styles from the past fifty years, as well as some from the future.

The atmosphere in the main-stage arena was unbelievable. Everyone seemed so happy, which really pleased me. I was so glad some of my special guests, like my friend Roberto Di Matteo, the fabulous football player-turned-manager who led my beloved Chelsea to win the European Champions League, were with me. Even more important, my wife Pauline was there with me to witness a wonderful evening, even if she did have her hands full, taking charge of some of my lively grandchildren!

The entertainment was absolutely stunning as Beardyman, Iggy Azalea, Labrinth and Tinchy Stryder all performed brilliantly. Sacha chose the Band of the Grenadier Guards to bring the fashion show to a fantastic climax in a wonderfully appropriate touch, which was really appreciated by everyone.

It was a fabulous way to celebrate our first half-century. As Sacha said, no other hairdressing company in the world has put on a show like this and I don't think they ever will. Toni & Guy is a special family with a special business but I want to remind everyone that although we have come a long way on our journey, deep down I felt one thing more strongly than anything else: we really have only just begun, *the next fifty years are going to be great!*

Celebrating our half-century worked wonders with my energy levels and 2014 has felt like I've been starting all over again. We certainly have a lot to feel good about. We reached our tenth year as the official sponsors of London Fashion Week. We obtained Superbrand status for the sixth year running, and Coolbrand status for the fourth consecutive year. Mainstage was a magnificent evening at The Copperbox, Olympic Park, which proved to be a wonderful new venue.

We've opened many more new salons in countries from Cambodia to Morocco and from India to Spain. Next year we're going to open up in Mongolia. That should be interesting. We had a fascinating visit to the United Arab Emirates where Sheikh Sultan bin Khalifa al Nahyan invited me over personally and was gracious enough to hold a dinner in my honour. He even introduced me to falconry! I have been invited to open a new hairdressing and beauty wing at Nottingham University. One of my next trips is for the salon opening in Casablanca, where we'll be staying in the former royal palace.

I have even found time to introduce my very own pasta sauce. It's made 100 per cent from Italian tomatoes from San Marzano and I am very proud of it and I hope everyone will enjoy it. Retirement? I haven't got time to even think about it!